THIRD EDITION

D1329382

Dancing

WITH

Dementia

SUCCESS WITH

SUPPORTIVE THERAPY

Len Fabiano

Dedicated To:

Linda

My wife, partner, best friend and confidant. Every accomplishment I have made is because of your love and support.

Acknowledgments

It is through the struggles of so many of the mentally impaired elderly I have known, that I learned of their experience; through the pain of so many families in their attempts to cope, that I learned of the need; and through the hopes and energies of so many professionals, that I learned what to do. To all of you my appreciation.

Likewise, there is a team of individuals who behind the scenes make my accomplishments materialize. To Nancy Cruickshank, Lloyd Dove and Pam White I thank you for your help, support and energy.

Len

CONTENTS

Chapter One

The Dance

There is nothing more majestic than professional ballroom dancing. Watching a couple in complete unison, matching each other's steps, moving as though they are one. One leads, the other follows in perfect harmony.

Caring for dementia clients with challenging behaviors is also a dance. The client leads. Each time we are out of step, the behavior is expressed. When we follow the client's lead and dance in unison, in step with the client, the outcome is positive for all.

Defining the Step

Dancing or caring for a dementia client with challenging behaviors involves complex steps. The complexity is created by two basic issues associated with dementia - the progressive brain damage caused by the disease process, and the increasing and ever changing sensitivity to stimuli and environmental factors.

The destructive nature of the diseases causing dementia can result in the brain shrinking up to 40% in weight and size. The progressive nature of the disease means that the client's abilities and needs are always changing. New symptoms can develop with little warning, existing symptoms will become more intense and complex, past symptoms will disappear. This ebb and flow creates a unique rhythm. If we are not in step, unable to identify what is happening, unable to assess the changes, unable to define the appropriate supportive measures and communicate them to all caregivers then the behavior will only intensify.

.

But the complexity of the dance continues. As the disease progresses and the symptoms change so will the individual's vulnerability to the stimuli around him. Many external factors influence this individual's behavior. When they are not understood, when what distresses him is not assessed, and the needed supports are not implemented, his behavioral response will only intensify. To be out of step with a dementia client with challenging behaviors will always create negative results for all.

The concepts presented in this text are based on Supportive Therapy. Supportive Therapy is a behavior management modality developed to respond to the destructive process of the disease and the associated areas of sensitivity to stimuli and environmental factors. The three principals associated with Supportive Therapy are:

1) Identify the individuals strengths and maintain them.
2) Identify the individuals limitations and compensate.
3) Identify the areas of vulnerability and intervene.

The first two principals address the progressive destructive nature of the disease, the third principal addresses the areas of sensitivity that must be controlled. Supportive Therapy allows the caregiver to dance gracefully with the dementia client demonstrating challenging behaviors, to move with the disease, to adapt to the changes, to continually stay in step.

Dementia Care versus Behavioral Management

The Supportive Therapy definition for Behavior Management as it applies to those with dementia is as follows:

An attempt to control the factors that have created and further complicated the person's life in order for the person to maintain their original self.

The first part of the definition 'factors that have created and further complicated the person's life' refers to the three principals of Supportive Therapy - maintaining the strengths, compensating for the limitations and intervening on the areas of vulnerability. The second part of the equation 'to maintain their original self addresses the quality of life issues as it pertains to their pre-morbid personality (who they were before the dementia).

It is important to understand the differences between behavior management and dementia care. These can best be demonstrated by comparing general duty nursing with specialized nursing practices.

The training in a general nursing program focuses on fundamental nursing practices. A nurse is trained as a generalist, equipped to care for a variety of needs presented by the typical patient. However, nurses in specialty areas like intensive care, psychiatry, emergency, etc., require additional training to ensure that their knowledge, skill set and practices match the needs of that specialty. No specialty nurse can be effective without the fundamental skills of the general duty nurse, and no general duty nurse can be effective in any specialty without specialized training.

Dementia care and behavioral management have the same symbiotic relationship. Dementia care provides the fundamentals of caring for those with dementia, a generalist approach on how to assist dementia clients to meet daily requirements and maximize quality of life, i.e. maintaining functions such as dressing, bathing, eating, participating in leisure activities, interacting with others, etc. Behavior management on the other hand involves specialized practices to address the challenges presented by:

- *high risk clients* - dementia clients demonstrating behaviors that can cause personal injury, such as elopement, wandering, ingestion of foreign substances, etc.

- *disruptive behaviors* - dementia clients demonstrating behaviors that have the potential to distress or agitate others, such as agitation, rummaging and hoarding, repetitive behavior, sexual behavior, etc.

- *high risk behaviors* - dementia clients demonstrating behaviors that have the potential to injure others, such as aggression, violence, aggressive wandering, sexual aggression, etc.

Programming is an excellent example of the differences between behavior management and dementia care. Dementia care programming applies to the majority of those with dementia and intended to entertain and occupy time. Behavior management programming is client specific and used to decrease the frequency, intensity and/or duration of a behavioral response.

These two modalities go hand in hand. Caregivers skilled in dementia care practices are not necessarily equipped to address challenging behaviors without behavior management training. Caregivers skilled in behavior management practices must be well versed in dementia care.

There are three levels of behavioral management: behavior care, behavior management and behavior crisis management. The definitions of these levels are as follows:

Behavioral Care - The potential for challenging behavior exists, however proactive measures result in acceptable expression of the behavior (no risk to self/others and/or will not initiate challenging behavior from others), or the behavior is not being expressed.

Behavior Management - The challenging behavior is expressed creating a potential risk to self/others, or initiates challenging behavior from others, however when specific care measures are employed the behavior returns to an acceptable level or is no longer expressed.

Behavior Crisis Management - The challenging behavior is out of control creating a high risk to self/others and requiring immediate resolution utilizing dramatic measures.

The three levels of behavior management can best be described by comparing them to the management of any disease. Take diabetes for example. The primary objective when treating diabetes is to administer a medication and provide a specialized diet that will stabilize the disease. When successful the person lives a normal life and others are often not aware that the individual has diabetes.

However, symptoms can develop either because the disease has worsened or the person does not follow the prescribed diet or take the required medication. In that case the care team will become more aggressive in their treatment, increasing the insulin or revising the diet, and providing more intense health teaching to ensure the patient follows what is required. The goal for this level of treatment is to eliminate the symptoms and return the individual to a stabilized state.

Unfortunately, it is also possible for the diabetes to become so severe, or the person to chronically not take his medication or follow his diet, that it is difficult to manage the disease. In this case high risk symptoms may develop requiring dramatic intervention, i.e. amputation of the person's leg due to complications.

The same progression is incorporated when caring for those with challenging behaviors. The first step is behavior care, implementing proactive measures to prevent a behavioral response. This requires specific assessment and analysis tools, as well as programming and environmental practices. When the behavior is prevented, there is no risk to the individual or those around her, no need for psychotropic medication, and individuals in contact with this client are unaware that the client has the potential for high risk behavior.

However, the progressive nature of the disease will produce new symptoms or intensify existing ones that can lead to an intense behavioral response; and/or the individuals sensitivity to specific stimuli within his environment can change also resulting in a behavioral response. When high risk behaviors are expressed then there is a need for more specialized tools. These are the complex practices of behavior management. These practices are intended to return the client to a managed state.

Despite these efforts, there may be times and circumstances when behavior crisis management is required. This is when a high risk behavior is out of control, placing the individual and/or others at risk. The primary recourse in this situation involves more dramatic measures (i.e. heavily sedating the client) in order to eliminate the risk for the client and/or others. Once the behavior is controlled, behavior management tools can be used to determine the cause for the behavioral outburst and define the course of action to prevent a reoccurrence.

Although this later case is not desired, intense behavioral responses can usually be avoided if behavior care and behavior management practices are in place. However, when behavior care or proactive practices are not practiced the situation is different. Return to the diabetes example.

Although the following scenario would never take place when treating diabetes, imagine the results if insulin was not ordered and a specialized diet not prescribed. The diabetes would progress unchecked causing a variety of serious symptoms. Once these symptoms occurred, then treatment would require substantial doses of insulin and a highly restrictive diet to stabilize the disease and eliminate the symptoms. However, once the symptoms are abated and the diabetes is stabilized, the insulin and diet are discontinued. If this cycle should continue (treatment then discontinue treatment) then the disease would eventually worsen to the point where dramatic measures are necessary (i.e. amputation of a leg due to complications).

Although individuals would be appalled if diabetes were treated in this way, this scenario can apply to how dementia clients with challenging behaviors are treated. When behavior care or proactive measures are not employed as a regular practice, frequent behavioral outbursts will result. When a high risk behavior occurs, the care team is often encouraged to implement behavior management practices, specialized tools to address high risk behaviors. However, without the skill and knowledge of performing behavior care practices or preventative measures, it will be impossible for the care team to be effective when required to implement more sophisticated complex practices. This results in the behavior management practices having little affect. Even if the behavior management practices did work to manage the behavior, they will provide only a temporary reprieve. The absence of preventative measures would result in the behavior returning. This cycle (treatment, discontinue treatment) would eventually leave behavior crisis management as the only recourse - to control the behavior with sedation. Once controlled, there would be little motivation on the part of the care team to remove the sedation when they have no alternate practices to fall back on to prevent the behavior from reoccurring in the future.

The scenario can become even more restrictive. Return to the case of diabetic treatment. No physician would withhold ordering insulin and a specialized diet, wait for the diabetes to be out of control and then simply amputate a patient's leg. However, that is not always the case in managing dementia behavior. When there are no behavior care or behavior practices available to caregivers, they can only wait for the behavior to become out of control and then sedate the individual in order to manage the situation.

Withholding treatment of a diabetic patient and simply amputating the individual's leg when the situation became severe would be considered negligence. Waiting for a dementia client to become out of control requiring dramatic measures (heavy sedation and/or physical restraining) should also be considered negligence.

Yet that is the case when behavior care practices or proactive measures are not entrenched within the culture of care. Without ongoing preventative measures:

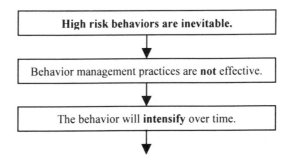

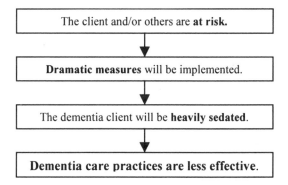

At first glance, behavior management appears to be caregiver centered not client centered, camouflaging the actual intent to manage the behavior for the caregiver's benefit. In actual fact behavior management is a highly intense client centered approach. It is based on a simple fact:

> *Behavior communicates a need.*
> *Addressing the need,*
> *Manages the behavior.*

All actions of Supportive Therapy are developed to decrease the stressors that trigger a behavior or adapt the care environment to meet the strengths and limitations created by the disease. When these factors are not controlled, the client becomes distressed and the behavior is expressed. To manage the behavior is to lessen or eliminate the impact of the causative factors.

"Dancing with Dementia" is about behavior care practices, addressing the causative factors to decrease or eliminate the behavior. The first step in caring for dementia clients with challenging behaviors.

The Road to Professionalism

Imagine a cardiac intensive care unit where the staff are not trained in cardiac care, CPR (cardiopulmonary resuscitation), do not have a cardiac monitor, stethoscope, blood pressure cuff, crash cart or any of the other specialized equipment necessary for a such a unit. The care staff are simply left to their own intuitive ability. It is obvious that staff would be unable to perform nothing more than basic care, only knowing when a patient is in distress when the signs and symptoms are so obvious that the patient's life is at risk. Even if a cardiac intensive care specialist were involved at this time there would be little that person could do given the severity of the problem encountered.

> Would you want your mother on such a unit if she experienced serious cardiac problems requiring specialized care?

In this case, the organization housing this unit would be considered derelict in their responsibilities and held accountable for any consequences that may result.

The same comparison can be made in caring for those with challenging behaviors. Without specialized training, assessment and analysis tools, specific programming and environmental options, specialized communication tools, etc. caregivers are left to function from an intuitive level only. They can only wait until the behavior is obvious and requires dramatic intervention (usually medication and physical restraint) to resolve what was more likely preventable. Even when a behavior management specialist is asked to consult, there is little this person can do at this time to manage the behavior other than recommend sedation. The ultimate consequences suffered by the client are obvious.

> Would you want your mother on such a unit if she had dementia and experienced challenging behaviors requiring specialized care?

Take this one step further. Imagine a cardiac intensive care unit where the staff are thoroughly trained and the equipment is state-of-the-art. A patient has a cardiac arrest. A caregiver runs for the crash cart and asks a co-worker for help. The comment from the co-worker is "I am going for coffee." It is difficult to conduct CPR successfully without help. Without assistance the patient will probably die. When the physician and family ask why the patient died, the only response is that a staff member ignored the cardiac arrest and went for coffee. Undoubtedly, the caregiver who went for coffee and ignored the cardiac arrest would be considered derelict in the performance of his/her duties and held accountable.

Yet, in some care settings, when a dementia client is in difficulty and a caregiver needs assistance to *prevent* an intense behavioral response, some caregivers will simply go for coffee and ignore what is required. The behavior would be expressed and sedation administered as a result. Yet, in those care settings, the caregiver who went for coffee and ignored the potential behavior would *not* be considered derelict in the performance of his/her duties nor held accountable.

Behavior Management is creating a major cultural shift in many health care organizations. The shift is to implement alternatives to dramatic measures (use of chemical and physical restraints) to manage challenging behaviors. A growing expectation of professional conduct by the organizations responsible for the safety and well being of these clients, and the caregivers who provide the care. An expectation that the organization will provide the needed training, tools and resources to properly manage this dementia clients with challenging behaviors. As well as an expectations that caregivers will no longer be allowed to ignore the needs of this client or refuse to implement appropriate practices without being held accountable for their actions regardless of their position or title.

Some organizations will argue that they do not have the resources to train their staff and develop these practices, and some caregivers will argue that they do not have the time to perform them even if they were in place. There is no argument that the resources available to organizations caring for dementia clients with challenging behaviors (both long term care facilities and community based programs) are strained. However, time and costs are a constant regardless whether these practices are implemented or not.

When these practices are not entrenched within the care culture or practiced by individual caregivers, then intense behavioral responses are commonplace resulting in:

- more time required by the care team to complete simple care tasks with these individuals, i.e. mealtime, washing, etc.
- usually more than one caregiver required to complete complex care tasks, i.e. bathing or dressing the client.
- a higher incidence of falls, incontinence, elopement behavior, client to client altercations, etc, requiring caregiver time away from scheduled care routines, increasing time pressures to complete regular duties.
- other clients becoming agitated by those with challenging behaviors, requiring additional attention by caregivers.
- a higher caregiver injury rate, increasing compensation and sick time costs.
- staff performance and retention problems caused by employee frustration and dissatisfaction with their work setting.
- higher costs and time demands to rectify resultant legislative infractions (i.e. increased incidence of client injury, elopement, medication use, etc.)
- a higher liability risk should injuries occur.
- the time demands to address family complaints regarding the care of their family member with challenging behaviors.
- the time demands to address family complaints regarding the influence of those with challenging behaviors on their family member.
- the loss of volunteers who are afraid or uncomfortable with those with challenging behaviors.
- a decrease in competitiveness (reluctance to admit due the behaviors witnessed during a tour of the facility; or due to the reputation of being unable to manage such behaviors.)

The difference is not time and cost, they are constant regardless of the steps taken. The difference is problem solving (implementing behavior care practices) versus crisis intervention. Crisis intervention is waiting for the behavior to be out of control. The costs associated with that choice are too high for all concerned. Health care organizations cannot afford "not to" implement behavior care practices, and caregivers cannot afford the time and subsequent risks "to not" use those practices.

Reading The Book

Regardless of what you do or where you work it is important to read the entire text. The tendency to skip sections because they appear to be site specific is to miss the significance of the information provided. The book has been written with two objectives in mind:

1) To assist individual caregivers regardless of their professional training and the location where they perform their care.
2) To assist organizations to develop the needed practices.

1) Individual Caregivers
The individual reader responsible for the care of dementia clients with challenging behaviors (whether family or professional caregiver) should not just read this book. The content and writing style is intended to challenge the reader to:

- define the rationale behind specific behaviors.
- validate what you are doing.
- examine your own care practices.
- provide you with a range of practice options.
- demonstrate the significance and value of certain practices to address specific care issues.
- learn methods to determine what should be done and when.
- provide ways to measure results and communicate them to others.
- assist in developing necessary safe guards and protective measures.

Examining the content in this way will allow you to expand and formalize your own behavior care practices in order to enhance your performance and success with those under your care.

2) Organizational Development

The second objective is to assist health care organizations to develop a Behavioral Care Practices Manual. The purpose of a practices manual is to provide all caregivers within that organization with the direction on what is to be done for this clientele to ensure consistency in performance and results. The components of a practices manual are as follows:

> *Foundations for Care*
> *Admission*
> *Assessment*
> *Analysis*
> *Programming*
> *Environment*
> *Family/Caregiver Support*
> *Outcome Measurements*
> *Behavioral Reference Section*

Each chapter outlines the content for a performance manual with the final chapters providing direction on how to develop a site specific manual and related performance audits to monitor the outcomes achieved.

Family, LTC, Acute Care, Community

The challenge facing this book is to address the needs of all who are responsible for the care of dementia clients with challenging behaviors, including family caregivers, long term care, acute care and community support programs. Each are similar and dissimilar in their responsibilities and challenges.

The similarities lies in the fact that the concepts causing the behavior are the same regardless of the setting and all are responsible to minimize challenging behaviors. The differences are as follows:

Family
Most family caregivers caring for a family member with dementia are exposed to a completely new and foreign experience. Challenging behaviors experienced by family caregivers can occur for one of two reasons:

1) The family does not understand the disease nor how to provide the care and supports, creating challenging behaviors (usually aggression, wandering or elopement).
2) The disease has progressed to a point where challenging behaviors are a result of the symptoms experienced.

The information and tools identified within this book are valuable for family caregivers. They will help to eliminate the external factors that may be causing the behavior. However, when the disease has progressed to the point where family are no longer able to address the behavioral demands (despite the efforts of community support programs), then placement to a long term care facility may be required.

Family cannot wait for the health care provider to uncover what is needed. Learning what causes the behavior and understanding behavior care practices allows family caregivers to create their personal practices manual as it applies to their family member. This allows the family caregiver to be an effective advocate by providing specific guidelines for anyone to replicate the care practices required, whether care is provided by another family member, by a community support caregiver assisting you in your home, or during a short stay in an acute care hospital, or permanent admission to long term care facility.

Community Support Program
Community support experience unique challenges:

- Often there is infrequent and short contacts with the client and the family caregiver.
- There are usually different community workers involved with the same case.
- There is little opportunity for community workers to come together to discuss a case.
- There is a need to know and replicate the care and approaches by the family caregiver.
- There is reliance on the family caregiver to follow-through on the practices developed by the community support workers.

A behavioral care practices manual ensures that all community workers are consistent in their performance, and provides family guidelines and interpretation of practices performed by the community support worker to allow replication of care.

In the event that the client is transferred to acute care or long term care, the practices manual and related information on the specific client will allow replication of care in those settings and provide family a way to advocate for consistency in performance.

Acute Care
The challenges facing acute care (i.e. emergency, ICU, medical and surgical units,) are at two levels:

1) The need to replicate the specific care practices developed by family caregivers, community support or long term care.

2) The challenges of conducting an intrusive or invasive threatening act (i.e. medical tests, surgery, specialized medical treatment, medications, etc.) with any dementia patient to.

If behavior care practices regarding a specific patient are not quickly learned and replicated, then introducing any intrusive or invasive threatening act will result in an immediate high risk behavioral response. Even if practices are replicated, the potential to experience an intense behavior response may still occur as a result of an intrusive or invasive threatening act.

A Behavior Care Practices Manual is necessary for all involved with this type of patient. It identifies information about how to care for this dementia client and what to do with any dementia client responding poorly to intrusive or invasive acts.

Long Term Care
The challenges facing long term care are even more intense:

- Long term care facilities are guaranteed to have many dementia residents demonstrating challenging behaviors.
- The mixture of these individuals, with cognitively well and higher functioning dementia residents can be volatile if the behaviors are not managed.
- The responsibility to care for these residents for the remainder of their lives means that caregivers will be subjected to countless changes in this resident's functioning ability requiring continual adaptations to the care practices being performed.

A practices manual defines how procedures, policies and practices are adapted for this client, and enhances consistency in performance. A practices manual is not only valuable for the caregivers within the facility, it accompanies transfers to acute care so they can replicate care practices for that individual. It also defines what is required from family caregivers and community support caregivers when a dementia client is admitted so that past care practices can be replicated.

Imagine the results if all four groups possessed a similar practices manual that could be shared from site to site. Moving the client from one location to the other would be made with minimal stress.

About the Book

The concepts and tools presented in this text have been field tested and practiced in scores of organizations, as well as presented in training seminars to hundreds of thousands of caregivers of varying levels of expertise. The modality is called Supportive Therapy. Supportive Therapy involves behavior management practices used with dementia clients presenting challenging behaviors and developed with the realities of the long term care industry in mind.

Do not be fooled by the practicality of what is presented. Any successful modality is one that can be replicated. The easier it can be replicated the more successful it will be. There are many years of research invested in the development of these tools with a dovetailing of each component to create the desired measurable outcomes.

The original book on Supportive Therapy was called "The Tactics of Supportive Therapy." It was highly successful and followed by a second book expanding on the concepts and practices. The sister book was called "Preventing Alzheimer's Aggression: Supportive Therapy In Action." The two books became popular with professional and family caregivers.

What was in the original book was suitable for its time. However, the research on dementia and the performance expectations of the health care industry have not remained stagnate. The knowledge about the diseases creating dementia has grown exponentially. Likewise, the health care industry serving this client has experienced significant changes:

- care based on defined measurable outcome.
- increased scrutiny of care practices by family members and the community at large.
- stringent legislative and legal requirements.
- vigilant client rights and advocacy requirements.
- increased safety expectations.
- competitive atmosphere by the private and public sector vying to service this growing market.

"Dancing with Dementia" is in response to these changes.

Parts of the original book "The Tactics of Supportive" are within this text. The basic concepts regarding the disease, experience, areas of vulnerability, symptoms, etc., have not changed. Likewise, original

Supportive Therapy behavior care tools still in use are also included. Of course sections from the original text have been edited, updated and/or condensed and new material, additional tools and concepts have been added.

The Content

The book has been divided into four sections

    Section One: Understanding the Client
    Section Two: Behavior Analysis
    Section Three: Behavior Care Practices
    Section Four: Specialization

The first three chapters within section one defines the uniqueness of this client and the foundation for a behavioral response. The first three chapters detail the experience, the disease process and the impact of secondary factors (areas of vulnerability). The next two chapters identify the contributors to a behavioral response and the challenges facing the caregiver.

Section Two is a comprehensive analysis of two common behaviors - wandering and sexual behavior. The intention of these two chapters is to demonstrate how behavior analysis is performed. These chapters identify the causes for each behavior and the subsequent supportive measures required to address each cause. The information provided in this section becomes the Behavior Reference Section of a Behavior Care Practices Manual.

Section Three outlines behavioral care practices. Individual chapters detail admission, assessment, analysis, programming and environment. The content of these chapters becomes the framework from which a practices manual is built. Also included in this section is an answer to a common question by caregivers, "What to say to a dementia client?"

Section Four focuses on specialization or developing a behavior care culture. This section involves a detailed description on the importance of a Behavioral Care Practices Manual, the required content and how one can be developed to be site specific. Also included in this section are Performance Audits. These are specific audits used to identify a care team's level of expertise and provide direction on areas requiring attention or development. Lastly is the concept of Modular care, creating specialized units and a detail Outcome Measurement Questionnaire. This questionnaire is an opportunity to evaluate the practices within your organization. The final section is the Addendum containing samples of assessment forms discussed within the text.

The Terminology and Focus

The terminology and focus of this book must be clarified.

Mental Impairment
Dementia will be interwoven throughout the book with another term - mental impairment. Mental impairment is used for two reasons.

1) Focuses on symptoms not diagnosis - Although Alzheimer's disease has the greatest visibility, there are many diseases that create the same clinical picture i.e. Lewy Body disease, Pick's disease, Creutzfield-Jacob disease, etc. Regardless of the diagnosis, the behavioral care practices presented apply to individuals demonstrating two basic symptoms - short term memory loss and loss of analytical ability or problem solving.

2) All mental functioning is involved - the term cognitive dysfunctioning is often misunderstood. Some believe that dementia causes a loss in thinking ability only. In actual fact, all mental functioning can be affected, including loss of physical abilities. Therefore the term mental impairment is used to encompass all mental abilities.

Mental impairment applies to any disease process that causes a deterioration in all aspects of mental functioning, and involves the symptoms of short term memory loss and loss of analytical ability.

Content Focus
Given that four groups require the information (family caregivers, community support programs, acute care and long term care), it is impossible to explain each concept, tool or practice as it applies to each specialty. Most of the material presented has a general writing approach that makes it applicable to any setting, however many of the case examples are predominately from a long term care perspective. This was intentional given that this client is common to that setting. Each tool in certain sections (especially assessment and programming) identifies the setting where it will have the greatest benefit.

Client
Likewise, the book cannot address the different terms used when addressing a person with dementia. For family the term is family member, for acute care it is patient, for community care it is client and for long term care it is resident. Client is the only universal term that can apply to all settings. It is important not to allow the neutrality of that term to depersonalize what is presented.

Beginning the Dance

Behavior care practices involve an investigative approach to care. Dementia clients do not have the ability to tell us directly what they require, however they will direct us to what is needed by their behavior. The caregiver must develop an intimate knowledge about the client in order to identify what is happening and determine what is needed. The effectiveness of any supportive measures is revealed by the client's response. If there is no change in the frequency, intensity and/or duration of the behavior, then the cause identified may not be accurate or the supportive measures not sufficient. If there is a change in the frequency, intensity or duration of the behavior then we are accurate in the direction taken. Your partner for the dance has been chosen. The lesson to help you follow your partner's lead will now begin.

Chapter Two

The Experience

There is a popular simulation that personalizes what it is like to be physically disabled, it is called, "Walk-A-Day-In-My-Shoes." In this simulation participants are given a mock disability. Some will have an arm tied to their body to simulate a stroke; others will have their fingers taped together to simulate arthritis; and still others, their eyes covered to simulate blindness.

Those who have experienced such a simulation usually report a dramatic effect - they move from thinking what it is like, to actually feeling what it may mean to be disabled for the rest of one's life. This is a very effective approach for caregivers to gain further insight into why a cognitively well, physically disabled client may withdraw or become aggressive under such circumstances.

How do you simulate dementia? There is no exercise that is as effective as the "Walk-A-Day-In-My-Shoes" simulation. Understanding how a dementia client may view her world is no easy task. The best that can be done is to compare this experience to something that may be common to many of us.

Being Lost

The following exercise involves a technique called Guided Imagery. Certain phrases are broken with a slash (/) to encourage you to pause and personalize what you have just read. Take your time and imagine the impact of each event.

Imagine:

You are walking through the woods sightseeing.

As the afternoon progresses you suddenly realize you are
   lost./
You are not sure which direction to go.
You experience a twinge of anxiety and fear./
You keep moving forward
Hoping to stumble onto something familiar.
You find that the further you go the more lost you become./
Hours pass, you are getting cold and hungry.
You know if you allowed it, the fear could intensify to an
   almost panic level./
As night time draws closer there is only one major priority-
   survival./

A person who is lost will experience five very distinct sensations.

- A constant anxiety that can easily turn into panic.
- The need to continually look for something familiar.
- Loss of peripheral vision.
- An egocentric behavior resulting in a loss of sensitivity to
   others.
- A fear for one's survival.

Anxiety to Panic - The first sensation involves a growing feeling of
anxiety and possibly even fear. These feelings require considerable
energy to prevent them from developing to a panic level. Surrounded
by this cloud of anxiety, rational thinking seems restricted as time
passes and the fear intensifies. Should that fear turn to panic and take
control, you could find yourself walking around in circles, passing the
same tree time and time again, and not even being aware of it.

Looking for Something Familiar - In conjunction with this anxiety,
you will find a constant urge or need to walk, always moving
forward. What motivates this action is a need to find something
familiar - a stream, a trail, a rock - something that will help you find
your way out. You know once you find something familiar, you will

be more in control of the situation and as a result your anxiety level will drop dramatically.

Loss of Peripheral Vision - In conjunction with this heightened level of anxiety and constant search for something familiar, there develops a further experience involving peripheral vision. While sightseeing, you will find your visual field is large and your visual ability quite acute. If during your walk there was a movement off towards your side you would have no difficulty noticing it, stopping to see if it was a deer or something else worth watching. However, when you are lost your peripheral or side vision wanes. The longer you are lost, the narrower your field of vision becomes. You develop what can be better termed narrowed or tunnel vision - concentrating straight ahead, looking for something that will help you find your way out.

Egocentric-like Behavior - Being lost also results in a person developing an egocentric-type behavior. If you and I were friends and lost together for a number of hours, how would you respond if I said to you: "I'm cold, I'm scared and I'm hungry"? Would you care? Probably not! It is difficult to worry about someone else's problems when you are experiencing the same thing yourself. This egocentric attitude results in our developing a very small internal world, one that at times involves our taking care of our own feelings and needs over the needs of others.

Survival - Lastly, there is a key word that will be experienced by those who are lost: survival. Am I going to make it through this?

These are the exact experiences of being mentally impaired.

Being mentally impaired is like being lost - living in a world that makes little sense. In such a state, it would seem that no matter what you did or where you went, you could not clearly make sense of what was around you. This can be demonstrated easily enough with your own clients.

Anxiety almost to panic - Imagine a confused and disoriented client who has lived within a long term care facility a year or longer. Even though that person may be mentally impaired, she has gained a degree of familiarity. She may not know exactly where she is, but she can find her room. She may not know staff by name, but she recognizes some by face. Place that same confused, disoriented client on a bus for an outing. The chances are good that while on that bus and during that outing her confusion will increase. We have now established one of the fundamental concepts involving the mentally impaired:

> *While moving from the familiar to the unfamiliar*
> *anxiety increases and mental functioning decreases.*

Family of a mentally impaired client will attest to this change in behavior. Moving a loved one from home to a hospital or long term care setting often results in a dramatic increase in that person's confusion and a decrease in his ability to accomplish tasks that were easily completed at home. Once a degree of familiarity is established within the new setting, the person will often regain the ability to perform many of those tasks once again.

Looking for Something Familiar - Many of the mentally impaired always seem to be looking for something familiar - house, spouse, clothing, etc. To look for something familiar in a world that does not make sense is an attempt to establish some control over the environment, which will in turn provide some sense of security and lessen the anxiety experienced. This constant search for something familiar explains why many mentally impaired individuals believe that:

- objects owned by others are their own, if they owned something similar to that in the past.
- people around them who have any similarity to family and friends (present or past) become those people.

25

Narrowing or Tunnel Vision - The third aspect that makes mental impairment similar to being lost is the change that occurs in one's peripheral vision. The mentally impaired experience a similar state of tunnel or narrowed vision.

The visual field of the mentally impaired can be compared to looking through a tunnel. They not only lose right/left visual acuity, but also visual acuity above and below eye level. The wandering client demonstrates this well. As we will discuss, there are two kinds of wanderers - the target wanderer and the aimless wanderer.

The target wanderer will commonly keep his eyes on his target. Should he turn away, his memory loss will likely result in his losing the knowledge of where he intended to go. However, the aimless wanderer, who will walk anywhere and everywhere, will generally keep her eyes down. If the individual is not looking down, she often trips over the simplest things.

This is a significant factor that dictates how a mentally impaired client is approached and how the environment must be planned (see the text "Preventing Alzheimer's Aggression," the Controlling Approach). If there is a need to hide something from a mentally impaired client, simply put it above eye level:

Out of sight is out of mind.

The following example demonstrates the impact of this loss of peripheral vision. A caregiver indicated that she was assisting a mentally impaired client with her shoes and socks while the client sat at the side of her bed. The caregiver said: "Initially the lady was so sweet saying 'Thank you dear. That is so nice of you dear.' Suddenly she hit me for no reason."

As we will demonstrate, in the majority of cases, that is not an accurate assessment of the situation. This example emphasizes the major concepts involving behavior care:

- There is a reason for every behavior.
- The dementia client always communicates, not necessarily verbally, but behaviorally.

- The individual's past history has a significant influence over present behavior.

Reason for Every Behavior - As we will identify, there is a reason behind the behavior of every dementia client. Discover the reason and you will identify what caused the behavior.

Always Communicate - Given that there is a reason behind every behavior, it is obvious that the behavior of the mentally impaired is always communicative. If you can read the behavior cues, you will gain considerable insight into what may be happening and the needed supportive measures. An effective behavior management tool is to re-create the events leading up to an intense behavioral response (see Behavior Incident Form under assessment). By re-creating the events it is possible to identify what triggered the initial behavior and determine the supports and interventions required to prevent further behavioral responses.

Re-creating the events leading to an intense behavioral response will provide direction on how to prevent the behavior in the future.

Past History influences Present Behavior - We know that the mentally impaired will lose short term memory and retain long term memory. In actual fact, they retain fragmented long term memory - pieces of the past instead of the entire memory. Past history influences present behavior. An important functional assessment question is to ask family to:

Identify significant events that stand out in your mom/dad's life for you as the son or daughter.

One thing that creates long term memory is emotion - whether positive or negative. It is easy to demonstrate. If you have children:

I want you
To go back in your past,/

27

To the first day/
You brought your first child home/
And all of the things that happened to you on that day./

When most remember that first day they smile. Can you remember what happened the seventeenth, twenty-second or thirty-first day after you brought your first child home? Probably not!

One of the things that creates long term memory is emotion. When an event elicits an intense emotional response, whether positive or negative, it will be easily imprinted in the brain and stored in long term memory. It does not matter whether the event elicits a positive or negative emotion. Do you still kick yourself now for a mistake you made fifteen years ago? All of us can relate to such an event.

In the case where the caregiver was struck by the client, she was asked if she knew this lady's history. The care team knew that this lady had been physically and sexually abused as a child and as an adult. The caregiver was then asked to demonstrate what she did at the time of the outburst (recreate the events leading to the behavioral response). The caregiver stated, "The client was sitting at the side of the bed and I was crouched down in front of her. She was watching me put her socks and shoes on her feet. Then I reached for one of her socks and she hit me." I then asked, "Where were her socks?" The caregiver replied, "On her bed to the <u>side</u> of her."

It became obvious that as long as this client could see the caregiver's hands, she felt comfortable with what the staff member was doing. As soon as the staff member reached to the client's side and beyond her field of vision, the client could no longer see her hand. Once the caregiver's hand was no longer visible, she was confused by that person's actions. This made her feel out of control, pushed her anxiety level to a panic state, and she became aggressive.

(This progression of events is called *The Aggressive Cycle* and described in the text "Preventing Alzheimer's Aggression: Supportive Therapy in Action" by Len Fabiano)

In this case, the care team was instructed that when caring for this client they must ensure that the client can see their hands at all times. This simple intervention resulted in a substantial decrease in this client's aggressive outbursts.

Egocentric-like Behavior - The fourth issue involves the egocentric-like behavior experienced by those with dementia. This is the inability to respond to the needs or feelings of those around. In counseling spouses of those with dementia, they frequently express concerns over what they witness: "My husband and I have been married for over forty years. During that time if I was ever sick, he would be there to help me every chance he had. If I was hurting emotionally, he would always hold me. Ever since he developed Alzheimer's, it never matters how sick I am, he doesn't help. Nor how much I am hurting, he never holds me."

It becomes almost impossible to be aware of what someone else is experiencing when you cannot deal with what you are going through yourself. As a result, the mentally impaired seem to be drawn into their own world and are oblivious to the feelings of others. They have lost the analytical ability to read the cues indicating when the caregiver is frustrated, busy or tired. They are also too overwhelmed by their own fear and emotion to be able to respond. When a dementia clients wants something, they want it now regardless of the needs of the caregiver.

Survival - Lastly is the element of survival. The main priority when encountering such a circumstance is to determine how to exist in a world you cannot understand. The dementia client must use whatever limited cues and information that makes sense to them, in order to establish some degree of control over what they are experiencing. They will attempt to make sense of that world to the best of their ability in order to survive.

This experience is not yet complete. Return to the scenario of being lost in the bush.

Shortly after you become lost
I appear./
You have never seen me before./
During the entire time you are lost
I stay forty steps behind you./

You walk forward,
I follow you./
You walk towards me,
I go the other way./
When you try to speak to me,
I do not answer./

How would this situation make you feel?

When you have a great deal of anxiety, if a stimulus appears that you do not understand, your mind goes crazy - "What does he want? What is he after?" Such an experience would undoubtedly intensify your anxiety level dramatically. Now your energies are not only concentrated on finding your way out, but trying to analyze my actions as well. It is amazing how poorly we can analyze an unknown stimulus when our fear or anxiety level is high.

Return to the simulation of being mentally impaired and a client in a long term care facility.

As a staff member
I have been in your room
Performing care from 0730 hours until 0800 hours./
At that time I left and returned again at 0845 hours
To take you to the bathroom./

Would you remember me? Given that you experience short term memory loss and cannot remember faces, probably not!

I walk to your side,

While standing next to you I ask,
"Do you have to go to the bathroom?"
Without any other direct contact or cueing,/
Would you know who I am talking to or what I am saying?

Highly unlikely! This scenario demonstrates another basic concept involving the mentally impaired:

> *If the stimulus is not intense enough,*
> *it will be missed (not seen or heard)*
> *or misinterpreted.*

When I asked if you had to go to the bathroom in the manner described above, you probably would not answer.

I then take you by the arm
And attempt to stand you up./
You would undoubtedly respond to my actions by resisting and
    becoming aggressive./

This experience can be called *Reality Shock*. My actions are faster than your thought process. Taking you by the arm without further warning requires you to instantly analyze where you are, who I am and what I am doing. You do not have the cognitive ability to respond that quickly. What you experience is a total stranger pulling you from your chair. You are confused by my actions. You feel further out of control. Your anxiety is intensified to a panic level and you will probably become aggressive.

There is little difference between this encounter and the earlier scenario where I followed you through the bush while you were lost. In both circumstances an unknown stimulus was presented at a time when you were already experiencing considerable anxiety. Your only logical response under such circumstances would result in your becoming defensive or even aggressive (either physically or verbally) in order to protect yourself.

We have taken a significant leap into the world of the mentally impaired elderly. The concepts described above will be expanded in the following chapters. We are still not finished attempting to understand the challenges that face this clientele.

Chapter Three

The Disease

There is a tendency by some caregivers to want the diseases causing mental impairment to be packaged into neat answers and predictions. The biological changes, cause, effects, results, course, etc. of these diseases provide no such luxury. The reality is that there is probably more that is not understood about this type of mental impairment than we understand. This is not a criticism of the researchers, but an emphasis on the challenges presented when caring for the mentally impaired.

It is important to stress that the diseases causing mental impairment are highly unpredictable. Understanding what is happening to the brain and the person is speculative at best. At present, a disease like Alzheimer's can only be diagnosed by autopsy or by a process of elimination (ruling out every possible treatable disease by thorough testing). When nothing else can be found that could cause the person's symptomology, then the conclusion is that it must be Alzheimer's. That, in itself, demonstrates the uncertainties these diseases present.

What complicates it even further is that we are not dealing with a disease process that is a separate entity of its own. There are many factors that influence mental functioning - emotional state, past intelligence level, past life history, effects of other diseases, drugs, sensory loss, etc. Combine any one or more of these factors with the unpredictable pattern of a disease like Alzheimer's, and you can clearly understand the challenges faced in attempting to define what is happening and what may happen.

Do not look here for neat, packaged answers about the disease process. The emphasis of this book is not on any one disease, but on effective care strategies. The information presented about the diseases causing mental impairment is intentionally condensed to ensure that a basic understanding of the biological process is established. This assures that the rationale for the supportive measures presented in the later chapters are understood. If further information is needed concerning medical research and theory, then it is important that one looks to other sources.

Understanding Alzheimer's disease

To demonstrate the biological changes that can occur, we will limit our discussion to only Alzheimer's Disease.

1) The Biological Changes

When most people think of damage to the brain at an older age, they often associate it with a dysfunction in the circulatory system. With Alzheimer's that is not so much the case. This disorder causes a dysfunction in the electrical conduction system of the brain, or how nerve cells or neurons within the brain communicate.

What seems to occur is a change in the manner in which messages are transmitted from one brain cell to another due to physical changes occurring in each neuron. The disease causes certain neurons to deteriorate, taking on a peculiar shape and eventually losing their ability to function.

Microscopic views of damaged neurons show nerve cells that "appear to be tied into knots." These configurations are called neurofibril tangles. At some point these cells are completely destroyed causing black patches of dead tissue throughout certain regions of the brain called senile plaques.

These changes can cause varying degrees of destruction and can be located <u>anywhere</u> in the brain. The predominant areas seem to be the temporal and frontal lobes, and the heart of the brain called the hippocampus. This presents an important consequence relevant to caring for those with Alzheimer's. The location and degree of damage is individualized. This dictates that no two individuals suffering from

Alzheimer's would be totally identical in the degree and location of destruction within the brain. Therefore, no two individuals will experience the same intensity and patterning of symptoms. As a result, behavior care practices are also individualized. What will work for one, may not work for another.

No two dementia clients experience the same
combination and severity of damage,
therefore care practices are highly individualized.

As a result, the challenges facing the caregiver are straight forward – there is no "cookbook" or universal way of caring for those with dementia. Each client presents a uniqueness that requires an individualized approach and program of care.

2) The Cause

At this time, the causes of diseases like Alzheimer's are unknown. Some have linked the changes in the brain to alterations in the genetic material of each cell, resulting in the cell virtually withering and dying from within. Others have associated it with the impact of a slow acting virus. Still others have linked it with the decrease in production of a neurotransmitter substance called acetylcholine, which is missing or in limited supply in the nerve cells of the brain. Still others . . ., the research continues.

3) The Effect

The most significant factor in Alzheimer's is the amount of damage done to the brain. Nerve cells within the brain are destroyed and lost. The loss of neuronal tissue can result in the brain decreasing in size and weight by as much as 40%. This one fact alone emphasizes the importance of philosophy when caring for those dealing with Alzheimer's:

What is lost is lost.

Alzheimer's disease is a progressive, deteriorating disorder which results in a progressive decrease in mental functioning until death (see Diagram #1). At present there is no way to cure or stop the disease. However, there are encouraging results in a new generation of medications that are intended to slow the progression of the disease and lesson the severity of some of the symptoms. Unfortunately little can be done medically to have a significant impact on the deterioration that occurs.

The destructive profile of the disease is significant in defining and evaluating any supportive measure. When a symptom or behavior is a direct result of the damage created by the disease, the practices are limited to supporting what is lost. This is the basic premise for the first two principles of Supportive Therapy; identify the person's strengths (what is still remaining) and maintain them, and identify his limitations (what is lost) and compensate for them.

This should not be surprising. This is the foundation for care with any individual experiencing brain damage. The expectations when caring for individuals with brain damage from a motor vehicle accident are obvious, we will:

- identify the areas of the brain that have not been damaged and encourage the person to maintain those remaining abilities.
- identify the areas that have been damaged and assist the individual in those areas.

There is only one difference when caring with those suffering from dementia:

we will identify the person's strengths and maintain them,
identify the person's limitations and compensate for them,
we will do that for the rest of the person's life
knowing only one thing will happen,
the individual will get worse.

We will always be required to adapt to the progressive nature of the disease – to continually "dance" with our client as his abilities change.

The Course of Alzheimer's disease

Alzheimer's disease can affect individuals as young as 40. It appears that the younger the individual, the more severe and rapid the deterioration. Like everything else with this disease there is no certainty, but the pattern seems to suggest that the <u>average</u> life expectancy of a younger person (the period from onset of the disease until death) is about two years.

The age group who more often encounters the disease are those over 60. The <u>average</u> life expectancy of an individual in this age group is about eight years, some living as little as two years and others as long as twenty years plus.

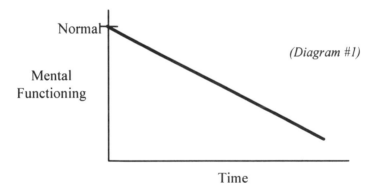

(Diagram #1)

It is difficult to pinpoint the exact duration of the disease for any individual. The onset of this disease is extremely insidious or slow. Given that the symptoms often develop gradually and initially can be easily hidden, accurately identifying when the deterioration began is no easy task.

It is important to emphasize the impact that the biological changes create. Areas of the brain that experience severe damage do not present the greatest challenges to the caregiver. The related symptoms are easily visible to anyone, regardless of their skills or abilities.

For example, if the area of the brain that recognizes names and faces is 90% destroyed, anyone within minutes of walking into that person's room would soon realize that this individual is unable to recognize people. The greater the severity of damage, the lesser the need for special skills or assessment tools to uncover what is lost. However, it is the *pinpoint areas* of destruction that create the greatest challenge.

The pinpoint areas of destruction represent the damage caused to small groupings of cells. Imagine the results if 90% of a certain area of the brain was still functioning, but only 10% was lost. If the caregiver does not possess the required assessment tools or specialized skills to identify the 10% that is lost, it will create considerable distress for the client. Let me demonstrate.

Imagine:

> I am mentally impaired./
> You give me my shirt,
> My pants,
> My socks and shoes.
> I get dressed with no problem./
> You put a pullover sweater in front of me
> I stare at it./

Those who do not understand the disease can mistakenly believe that my stalling to put on the pullover sweater is intentionally attention seeking or resistive behavior. That assessment would be wrong!

Each of us possess a cell in our brain that stores the picture of a pullover sweater, this allows us to do something called recall. We look at a pullover sweater, compare it to the picture in our brain and then know what it is and what to do with it. However, if the cells that store the picture of a pullover sweater are destroyed, then that type of sweater becomes a foreign object. We will react as though we had

38

never seen one before. This symptom is called Agnosia, the inability to recognize objects.

> *When certain cells or groupings of cells are destroyed,*
> *the memory or function stored within those cells is lost.*

Without the functional assessment tools to uncover these subtleties or a way to communicate this information to all in contact with this client, then the person may be pressured to perform something that she is unable to do.

Take this even further. An individual may be able to recognize a pullover sweater and even call it by name, but unable to identify the bottom, the top, the left or right. In this situation, the cells that store the imagery of what a pullover sweater looks like are intact. However, the area of the brain that allows the person to use the object is lost. That is the second component to agnosia: the inability to manipulate an object.

When this symptom was shared with a client during counseling, she started laughing. When asked why she was laughing she said, "My husband has the disease. He will ask for a pullover sweater or call it by name when he sees one, but he always puts it on like a pair of pants." You cannot help but admire the tenacity of the mentally impaired to make sense of something, even though they have limited ability and information. Not knowing what to do with the sweater once he sees one, he then functions to the best of his ability - to him, it has a waist, it has legs and it has a funny looking fly.

The damage within the brain can be even more refined. You pat the seat on a chair and say, "Please, sit on the chair." The client sits down. Twenty minutes later the person is walking past you and you ask him to sit down on the chair without physically directing him to a chair. The person does not respond. The reason is simple – he does not know the meaning of the word 'chair'. When he sees one he knows what it is and what to do with it, however he cannot remember what it is called. This is the third part of agnosia - the inability to associate words to an object.

This one symptom demonstrates the complexity of this disease. Agnosia can result in any one of the following three outcomes:

- inability to recognize the object or use it
- ability to recognize the object by name but not know how to use it
- ability to use the object but not call it by name.

Imagine the impact if a caregiver was unable to identify these strengths and limitations.

Pinpoint areas of destruction can occur throughout the brain. Identifying these areas and determining ways to adapt care is one of the primary focuses of Supportive Therapy. In order to discover the client's strengths and limitations, the caregiver requires a battery of functional assessment tools. The more diverse and varied one's 'bag of tools', the greater the chance to successfully adapt to the needs of the individual client.

Levels of Functioning

When discussing the mentally impaired, it is important to define the changes in functioning that can occur. We need to discuss three distinct levels of care. These levels should not be confused with the phases or stages of the disease. The stages of the disease describe the biological process that may be occurring. These levels define the person's functioning ability and the resultant care that is needed.

Level One

General Characteristics
- *Physically well.*
- *High functioning.*
- *Often living at home.*
- *Symptoms are a nuisance, easily compensated.*

- *Able to respond to programming and activities of daily living well with minimal supports.*
- *Major problem is mood swings.*
- *Undergoing intense grieving.*

These represent the initial effects experienced with the disease. During this time the individual may not be diagnosed. However, this individual is soon aware that something may be wrong, and often is unwilling to admit that it is anything serious.

In fact, at the beginning or onset of the disease, few who associate with this individual are even aware that there is anything seriously the matter. The symptoms are much too subtle and the progression too insidious to create alarm. It is only when the individual does something very peculiar that the family becomes concerned and seeks medical attention.

Imagine:

> I am 78 years old,
> Your father,
> Living with you in your home./
> We are sitting in your kitchen.
> I am attempting to balance my bank statement./
> I find I can't do it.
> It is not just the bank statement that is the problem,
> The numbers just don't make sense./
> A month ago I had little problem with this task.
> Now adding simple numbers seems impossible./
>
> Instead of expressing concern
> I innocently pass you the book
> Stating, "I can't seem to get this to balance with my cheques,
> Would you check it for me?"/

Father seems to always have a reason for his inability - he is overtired; it is too complicated; he just needs help; he is thinking about something else and cannot keep his mind on what he is doing; etc., an endless list of excuses. In actual fact, he is merely camouflaging his difficulties. Afraid or reluctant to admit that his "mind is failing."

Normally there is little alarm on the family's part - a 78 year old father having trouble making the bank statement balance is not unusual. In fact most of us experience that problem from time to time. Family are not quickly conscious of the recurring pattern of father's limitations. They simply attribute it to a slight forgetfulness or unfortunately stereotype his behavior as simply "old age." In actual fact, father has difficulty with all numbers.

To your spouse, he states - "I keep getting the numbers of your address mixed up with my old one at home. What are they again?" Or to one of the kids, "What's the last three digits of our phone number, it's slipped my mind again. And the first, and second? That's right!" Sounds more like he is correcting you than not remembering himself.

At this point members of the family are usually not alarmed. They do not collaborate and identify a pattern in dad's inability to function as he used to - only a 78 year old dad who is having some trouble remembering things. It is not until some peculiar behavior - wandering onto the street partially dressed - does the family become alarmed and take dad to the doctor.

Once the doctor has completed a thorough examination and ruled out any treatable cause for his impairment, he then makes the diagnosis of Alzheimer's disease. He will explain to the family the progression and characteristics of the disease. It is then that the family pull it all together, often exclaiming, "This may have been going on with Dad for years, but we didn't see it!"

It is not unusual for family members to question, "Had I brought Dad to the doctor two years ago when it first began, would it have made a difference?" The answer, of course, is no. There is no treatment for the disease or a way of curing it. Unfortunately some family members may not accept that response. They needlessly feel guilty for not doing something earlier, even though nothing could have been done to change the situation.

At level one, the person not only experiences an increasing degree of anxiety, but a considerable amount of frustration as well. This frustration arises from the fact that the person knows she could perform a certain task or easily remember things only a short while ago, but as time passes she finds it harder and harder to maintain those abilities.

An dementia client at level one requires little physical care, only specific supportive measures to address those things that present the greatest difficulty. In fact it is not the symptoms that create the problems as much as the associated emotions. This person demonstrates frequent and abrupt emotional swings that can create significant problems for family and professional caregivers.

Imagine how you would feel if you discovered or suspected seriously that you had Alzheimer's disease. You would go through every stage of the grieving process:

Denial: - "I am not sick, there is nothing wrong with me."
Blaming - "Why are people always hiding things on me."
Bargaining - "Maybe if I eat only certain foods or take vitamins
            or herbs I can make it better."
Depression - "I give up, there is nothing left for me to do."
Anger - "This shouldn't be happening to me."
Acceptance - "I must get on with what remains of my life."

Grieving is the response to any loss. As the disease progresses and the person's functioning deteriorates further, he experiences further loss in ability. At this level the person is fully aware of what he loses and responds accordingly.

Unfortunately, this disease does not remain static. It is always changing. A person at this level may initially begin forgetting the location of things. He looks for a cup in the kitchen. He starts at the first cupboard where he thinks it is. It's not there. His anxiety is increasing over his inability to find it. He goes to the second cupboard where he believes the cup may be, again it is not there. He becomes frustrated further. He goes to the third cupboard, it is still not there. Now he is very angry and slams the cupboard closed. Unfortunately, the cup is in the fourth cupboard he opens. By this time he is so angry with himself, he doesn't see it. He slams the cupboard closed, and moves to the next cupboard.

This demonstrates a significant fact in dealing with <u>any</u> mentally impaired client <u>regardless</u> of the functioning level experienced.

> *When a mentally impaired client loses control.*
> *mental functioning is lost.*

Had this individual just stopped, taken a deep breath and concentrated, he would have found the cups. When he lost control, he lost the ability to analyze stimuli and solve the problem that confronted him.

To prevent a person at this level from losing control, things cannot be left to memory. Therefore *cue cards* are used. These are small cards that are placed on cupboard doors, dressers and closet doors, listing by word and picture what is behind that door. This prevents the need to continually search to find the item. He simply reads the cards.

Unfortunately, many of my clients initially do not call these cue cards. They call them "idiot cards." To ask a 78 year old to use little cards like a two year old can be degrading, a major assault on one's independence and self image. It is another loss and will again initiate any or all of the stages of grieving.

Denial - "I don't need those things. I can find things when I want to."

Blaming - "If you would just put things where they belong, I wouldn't need these stupid cards."

Bargaining - "We'll put the cards up when I really need them."

Depression - "Put the cards up, it doesn't matter anymore."

Anger - "You put those cards up and it shows me that you don't love me."

Acceptance - "Fine, even though I don't like them I will use the cards."

Hopefully, after a period of time, he will understand the importance of such a supportive device. When he reaches acceptance, he will finally admit to himself that he can no longer function by memory to find the things he needs and will use the cards. Unfortunately, a few days later he cannot remember his daughter's name. That is a new loss. The grieving process and emotional swings will begin again. This explains why one day the person is their "old self," the next is withdrawn and despondent and the next is "taking someone's head off" at the slightest thing.

These emotional swings are the hardest for family and caregivers to deal with. In fact the wife will frequently complain, "Why does my husband always makes a scene, yet he doesn't want anyone to know he has the disease?" In this scenario, the husband attempts to act as "normal" as possible. However, when he loses control, he loses control of his emotions as well.

Imagine:

> You and I are married./
> I have been diagnosed with the disease.
> I do not want anyone else to know./
>
> We have company over for coffee.
> Everything is proceeding normally./
>
> I mention to our guests,
> "Did Mary tell you that last October
>   the basement flooded . . ."
> I proceed to tell our company an accurate account of the
>   details of that incident./
> Not five minutes after I finish
> I interrupt again by stating,
> "Did Mary tell you that last October
>   the basement flooded . . ."
> Again I recall the story in full./
> The company smiles./

Only five minutes later, I interrupt the conversation again,
"Did Mary tell you that last October
    the basement flooded . . ."
Telling the story at length once again./

The company stares at the ceiling or shakes their head./
When I notice their response
I get angry and pound my fist on the table./
I turn to you and yell,
"I am sick and tired of these people, don't invite them here
    again!"/
I storm out of the room./

In this situation the husband is not intentionally "making a scene," but responding to his loss of control. At this level he quickly forgets what he has just said, and frequently repeats himself. Unfortunately, his cognitive ability is high enough to enable him to read the non-verbal response of those around. Each time he sees them react, he realizes that he must have done something wrong, even though he does not know what it was. At that point he becomes angry with himself, loses control and lashes out at those around him.

A major concern for a client at this level is the possibility of suicide. The future can hold tremendous fear when a person is aware that he has the disease and knows what may be in store for him as it worsens. However, suicide attempts at this level may not be overt or obvious (hanging or by shooting). They may instead be covert or hidden - over-medicating one's self, falling down stairs, car accident, etc. With a car accident it only takes a second to decide, "I have had enough" and pull the wheel.

This is not intended to elicit undue alarm by family or professional caregivers. They should not overreact and read every act, conversation or incident as a desire to commit suicide. However, all aspects and effects of this disease must be discussed, even though they may be very painful or too difficult to admit.

This raises the issue:

> Should a person diagnosed of Alzheimer's disease be told
> he/she has it?

If a person had terminal cancer, would you tell that individual? If the answer is "no I wouldn't," it is unfortunate. How can you help a person overcome some of the symptoms if the person does not know what is happening? Supports are required to compensate for what is lost in order for the person to function at his/her maximum level. If you don't tell the person he has the disease, how do you place the cue cards around the house?

I remember a man in his late forties who sat in one of my presentations on Alzheimer's disease. He and his wife approached me at the end of the session and he told me he had just been diagnosed with the disease. I responded, "Whatever you want to say to your family or do to ensure that things are taken care of, you must do it now!" He responded, "You are scaring me!" I told him that he could not wait. With this disease, there is no way to predict what will happen and when. He needed to resolve issues while he was still able, as would any person who knew he would die soon. The realities of this disease demonstrates the harshness of its effects and the difficulties in coping.

In fact a common concern that I have frequently heard from those at this level is:

> *"It is not just the disease that scares me, but knowing that at*
> *some point during the disease I will no longer be in control of*
> *my own dignity, but must rely on others to control it for me."*

I have just revealed to you a personal commitment that I have made to those at this level of functioning, which is reflected continually in the concepts of Supportive Therapy -

> *A vow to respect that person's dignity*
> *regardless of ability.*

Level Two

<u>General Characteristics</u>
- *Physically well.*
- *Ambulatory.*
- *Very confused and disoriented.*
- *Main care challenges are behavioral.*
- *Has difficulty performing activities of daily living.*
- *All programming must be adapted to meet his specific level of mental functioning.*
- *Significant supports are required.*
- *The environment must be controlled to decrease the amount of stress and stimuli encountered.*
- *In contact with two distinct worlds, theirs and reality as we know it.*

A dementia client at this functioning level is often physically well, ambulatory, demonstrating considerable wandering and aggressive behavior and is very confused and disoriented. Mentally, this is an individual in frequent conflict. This person seems to be aware of two worlds existing at the same time - theirs and reality as we know it.

Imagine:

> I am mentally impaired,
> Living on your unit./
> Being disoriented
> I believe that I work here or am only visiting./
> At 3 p.m. staff head for the door to go home./
> I follow./

> When I reach the door
> One of the afternoon staff stops me,
> Stating, "Len, you have to stay, this is where you live."/
> I respond angrily,
> "I don't live here. I'm going home."

I fight to push past her./

This person's confusion and disorientation results in his not knowing where he is. He may believe that he is not a resident of a long term care facility, but only a visitor. When he sees staff leave to go home, he follows. Being stopped and told this is his home, causes him to be further confused. His confusion intensifies his feeling of being out of control. His anxiety elevates to a panic state, which results in his wandering or becoming aggressive. A person at level two has enough comprehension to know what is being said or is aware of certain aspects of what is happening, but what is said or happening is in conflict with what he believes.

In the upcoming chapters it will be frequently demonstrated that the world of the mentally impaired is real to them. Our challenge is to better understand that person's reality in order to adapt our interventions accordingly. It is those in level two of functioning that pose the greatest challenge to the caregiver.

A person in level two responds differently to surroundings and circumstances than level one. As demonstrated earlier, those in level one are still aware of the subtle cueing available in the environment. Level two does not have that degree of comprehension. As a result, his response to situations are dramatically different.

Imagine:

> You and I are married./
> I have been diagnosed with Alzheimer's disease.
> It has now progressed to level two./
>
> You have company over for coffee./
> I sit down and join you.
> Immediately I interrupt the conversation stating,
> "Last October the basement flooded."
> You respond, "Yes dear."/
> Two minutes later, I interrupt the conversation again,
> "Last October the basement flooded."

> You respond again, "You've just told us that."/
> "Yes, but the basement flooded."
> The company smiles./
> "Last October the basement flooded."
> The company stares at the ceiling and shakes their head./
> "Last October the basement flooded."
> Finally they excuse themselves and leave./

At this level the person is no longer capable of picking up the subtle cueing of facial expressions and body movements from those around to indicate that something is wrong. He has very severe memory loss and cannot remember what he just said as soon as he said it. He goes on repeating himself until he clears the room and even then may still continue.

The only time a person in level two of functioning may become frustrated and possibly be aggressive is if family continually tell him that he is repeating himself or try to stop him, rather than accepting his behavior. At this level, family no longer deal with the emotional outbursts experienced when the client is in level one. They must now cope with the repetitiveness of the individual's behavior and their own possible frustration in not being able to stop it.

This is not to suggest that a person at level two is oblivious to her environment. There are certain aspects of her surroundings that she will respond to and others that she cannot interpret or even perceive. This person is very vulnerable to her surroundings and the events that occur around her. The majority of this text is dedicated to understanding what an individual at this level may be experiencing and the necessary strategies required in his/her care.

Level Three

General Characteristics
- *Mentally and physically incapacitated.*
- *No longer able to walk.*
- *Incontinent.*
- *Limited awareness of their environment.*
- *Believed to be in a state of contentment.*
- *Generally unaware of surroundings except for very basic stimulus like touch, sound, voice tone, etc.*
- *Requires total care in activities of daily living.*

A person at this level of functioning is incapacitated both physically and cognitively. Physically this person requires complete care - being fed, washed, dressed and is totally immobile. Mentally this person seems oblivious to the world around her. She appears not to be aware of a person's presence until she is touched. Even then she probably does not understand the content of what is said or who is saying it. This person responds mainly to basic stimuli. If pulled roughly out of a chair or talked to in a loud and aggressive voice, she will instinctively jerk back or become afraid. Those in level three require total care and respond to limited programming.

Yet, it is the person in level three who best represents the cornerstone to the basic philosophy in effectively caring for the mentally impaired elderly.

Imagine:

Your mother is in a car accident./
She is admitted to an Intensive Care Unit in hospital.
She is totally unconscious and on all life supports./
As the ICU nurse,
How would you want me to treat your mother while she was
in that state?

The answer is obvious. Caregivers would be expected to treat your mother as though she could understand what was happening around her.

Only a small percentage of what is in our mind is at the conscious level. A much larger portion is in the unconscious. Even though a person at level three seems oblivious to what is going on around her, we do not know what that individual can see, hear, feel or understand. Given that fact, it is mandatory that:

> *We treat this person with the expectation*
> *that everything and anything can be understood,*
> *even though the person cannot indicate that is the case.*

The expectation of anyone in contact with the mentally impaired is to treat that person:

> *As a normal functioning adult,*
> *but not to expect normal behavior.*

It will be emphasized repeatedly in the following chapters that the way this person is perceived and treated will play a substantial part in how this person acts. If the mentally impaired is treated as a child, she will probably respond with child-like behavior. If she is treated as though she were "crazy," she will probably present "crazy-like" behavior.

There is nothing more irritating than to watch two caregivers standing over a mentally impaired client, talking about him as though he were not there. It is no wonder the person is agitated. Appropriate programming (what is required to ensure effective care) at this level can be compared to the concept of palliative care.

It is well known that when a person is dying and unconscious, it is extremely valuable for family or a caregiver to sit with that individual, stroking his hand and talking to him. Physical and emotional security must be provided regardless of a person's functioning level. When dealing with level three, it can only be communicated by the most basic of means.

MULTIPLE INFARCT DISEASE

A second very common condition causing mental impairment in the elderly is Multiple Infarct Disease (MID). This condition is a series of small strokes due to a dysfunction in the circulatory system of the brain. The difference between Multiple Infarct Disease and what is commonly known as a "stroke," is the lack of physical paralysis. The damage experienced in MID usually causes a dysfunction in mental ability only and the symptoms presented very much resemble those commonly encountered with Alzheimer's disease. What differs between MID and Alzheimer's is the course and the progression.

Unlike Alzheimer's disease, Multiple Infarct Disease can be very quick in its onset. When the individual experiences the first "stroke," obvious changes in cognitive functioning can be noticed.

Like any "stroke," the initial trauma or assault to the brain causes edema or swelling of brain tissue. This swelling can result in the victim demonstrating severe and multiple symptoms. As the swelling decreases over time, many of the initial symptoms may abate. This is often the case with a stroke. Individual's who experience total right sided paralysis may regain much of their functioning within only a few weeks. What may remain is a flaccid or limp right arm. The same is true of Multiple Infarct Disease. The severity and multiplicity of the symptoms may improve somewhat after the initial onset.

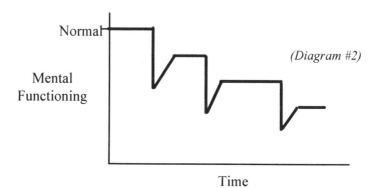

Normal

Mental
Functioning

(Diagram #2)

Time

What is significant about this disease is the potential for further strokes. When one cerebral infarct or "stroke" is encountered, the chances are high that another may be experienced. This step-down deterioration - stroke, loss in functioning, slight improvement, stabilizing for a period, then stroke, loss of functioning, slight improvement, etc. - may continue until death (see Diagram #2). Death is often caused by a major cerebral hemorrhage.

To demonstrate the course and progression of this condition, let us examine an actual case. We will call him John (age 69).

One Tuesday afternoon John sat in his favorite easy chair for a nap. When he woke half an hour later he was completely confused, disoriented and violent, striking out at family members who approached him. He was taken to hospital. Two weeks after his admission he improved considerably. His memory had returned, he was able to identify members of the family, he knew where he was.

The residual effect of the initial "stroke" was his inability to problem solve at a very basic level and loss of short term memory. From that point on, if he was asked to place a top on a pen he had considerable difficulty completing the task. He even had problems, at times, getting into a box of chocolates. All of his other faculties and abilities seemed to be functioning well.

The next month he experienced another cerebral infarct. It was very subtle, possibly showing itself as a slight dizzy spell or momentary blackout. It could even have happened during his sleep. Now he lost control over his emotions. He could not stop crying even though he stated that he felt fine. The next month he had a major hemorrhage which finally killed him.

The interventions employed in caring for an individual with Multiple Infarct Disease are the same as those for Alzheimer's - identify that person's strengths and maintain them, identify his limitations and compensate - Supportive Therapy.

Rather than investing further energies to expand the biological nature of the disease process, it is more important to identify what we as caregivers can do to assist the mentally impaired to live to their fullest. Many believe after learning about Alzheimer's and Multiple Infarct Disease and other such diseases that little can be done. On the contrary, much can be done. Curing or reversing the organic changes experienced by the brain is not possible, but providing individuals of such disorders the highest level of quality of life given the circumstances experienced is our main responsibility.

To determine the most appropriate living environment for any mentally impaired client requires that we define this person's vulnerability. The mentally impaired are sensitive to the world around them. Any mentally impaired client may experience further limitations in her functioning ability by external factors including inappropriate approach, an underlying disease process, a faulty drug profile and a confusing environment. Much can be done on our part to control each of these situations in order for each client to achieve his/her highest level of quality of life given his limitations.

Chapter Four

Secondary Factors

The sensitivity of the mentally impaired to external factors is a major concern for all caregivers. Secondary factors are external circumstances that further impair the individual's functioning ability. These vulnerabilities or sensitivities can be divided into four categories:

- Drugs
- Other Diseases
- Approach
- Environment

If any of these factors are not controlled, the cognitive ability of a mentally impaired client will decrease, further decreasing the person's mental functioning and performance (ability to complete specific tasks), and creating any one of a variety of behavioral responses. Diagram #3 demonstrates the potential change that can occur.

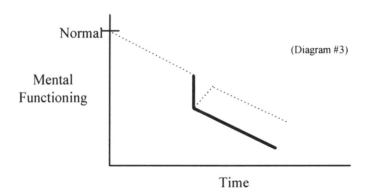

Normal

Mental
Functioning

(Diagram #3)

Time

The course of the disease is the dotted line. The sudden drop in the person's mental functioning level (solid line) can be the result of one of the above factors. Should the factor decreasing this person's functioning ability be removed, then the individual's functioning level, performance abilities and behavior would return to their "normal" state (dotted line): the level the client should demonstrate given the degree of brain damage caused by the disease process.

Secondary factors describe the up and down swings of ability, confusion and behavior experienced by those with dementia: why the person can perform one thing one hour and not the next; why the person behaves one way during one time of the day and another the next. It is important to emphasize that generally these shifts are not characteristic of the diseases causing dementia. Symptoms related to the progression of the disease are insidious or slow in their progression. Sudden shifts are more characteristic of secondary factors.

Drugs

The sensitivity of older people to medication has been a long standing concern. Aging creates specific biological changes that can alter bodily functions. These changes have the ability to affect the older person's response to many medications. Some of the major physical aging changes that can affect drug utilization are:

- a decrease in absorption of substances through the gastrointestinal tract.
- a slowing of metabolism or the breakdown of substances within the body.
- less effective excretion of substances from the body.
- alterations in the circulatory system in transporting substances within the body.
- changes in the location and amount of fat deposits affecting the storage of substances within the body.
- an increase in total body water weight.

The majority of these changes are gradual in nature and usually moderate in their degree. As a result, most older people do not experience any dramatic restrictions in their ability to function in their daily living activities. However, it is apparent that these changes can affect medication use by increasing the risk of a toxic level - even with therapeutic dosages.

Determining the most effective drug to treat a specific disorder experienced by an older person is not an easy process. What complicates it further is that physical changes caused by the aging process occur at different times, to a different intensity with each person. That makes it difficult to predict whether a medication taken by one older person would have the same impact on another. A toxic or adverse effect experienced by one older person to a specific drug does not mean that another will not be able to tolerate and benefit from that same medication.

This individuality in drug response is characteristic to the mentally impaired as well. Some medications work well with certain mentally impaired clients, while those same drugs at the same dosage have a devastating effect on others.

These discrepancies are complicated even further by the fact that the mentally impaired are significantly more sensitive to medication than the older population in general. This makes medication use with the mentally impaired a major concern.

The information on medication use and the elderly is growing, but information on medication effects on the mentally impaired elderly is limited. This lack of information makes it difficult to discuss specific brand name drugs when talking about their potential impact on the mentally impaired. In our discussion, specific examples can only refer to categories of medications rather than brand names themselves. Besides, it is not the specific drug that is important, but understanding the impact of any medication on any one mentally impaired person that is the issue. With any mentally impaired client, functioning on all counts can deteriorate dramatically given the wrong medication at the wrong time.

Sleeping medications or hypnotics are prime examples of this phenomenon. Certain sleeping pills have a devastating effect on the mentally impaired. One popular drug in this category has what is called a "100 hour half life" in some individuals over 65. (half life is the length of time it takes for half of one dose to be eliminated from the body.) In simpler terms this means if a 78 year old is sensitive to that specific drug it will take 100 hours for half of one dose to leave the body. Imagine the impact if that drug is given five nights in a row.

Giving the same sleeping pill to a mentally impaired client who is as sensitive would have devastating effects. To administer the drug five nights in a row would invariably mean that she will be unable to feed herself breakfast or dress herself in the morning. This change in functioning is not directly attributed to the disease process, but to her sensitivity to this secondary factor (diagram #3).

A similar effect can be encountered with almost every category of medication. Anti-anxiety agents are another example. Certain commonly used drugs in this group have a half life equivalent to age. This means when an 80 year old is sensitive to this specific medication, it can take up to 80 hours for half of that drug to leave the person's body. Some of these agents possess a six half life duration (the entire length of time for the drug to be totally eliminated from the body). That equates to 480 hours, twenty days for all of that drug to leave the body (the first 80 hours, half of the dose is lost, the second 80 hours, half of the half, etc.). The result is a highly toxic effect that decreases the person's ability to concentrate and perform many tasks.

The negative impact of certain medications on the elderly can be dramatic. We know little about the effect of one drug on an older person, let alone a combination of possibly five or more different medications taken in a twenty-four hour period. This sensitivity is compounded even further with the mentally impaired elderly. Their reaction to psychotropic medication (drugs used for behavior) may be as great as four times what is experienced by the older population in general. This makes medication use with the mentally impaired elderly a primary concern.

Whenever a mentally impaired client's behavior changes or functioning level deteriorates (whether physically, mentally or emotionally) the first questions that must be asked are:

What change has been made to the dose or times of medications
given?
What new drug has been ordered?

If a recent change in medication has occurred (anything within the
past month), then that should be investigated as its possible cause.

The sensitivity of any mentally impaired older person to
medication creates the need for ongoing assessment and a conscious
trial and error approach in medication usage (see assessment section -
Three Month Review and Trial Period Without):

- starting an older person on a specific medication.
- observing closely for side effects created.
- being willing to alter the type or dose of the drug should
  side effects persist.

In fact, the best philosophy with medication use and the mentally
impaired elderly is:

When in doubt, do without.
When in use, use the minimum.

It is important to clarify this statement. There are times where
psychotropic medication or drugs used for behavior are required:

- as a stop gap measure in order to define the most appropriate
  care strategies and supports to decrease the challenging
  behavior.
- when the behavior is directly related to the damage caused by
  the disease.

Other Diseases

Any acute or chronic physical disease or circumstance that alters
an individual physical state can decrease a dementia client's mental

functioning, increase confusion and decrease functioning ability. The organic changes experienced by the brain of a person with dementia or Multiple Infarct Disease can create considerable sensitivity to alterations in any body process. The brain's effectiveness to perform can be hampered by changes to any of the major organs of the body - liver, heart, lungs, circulatory system, kidneys, etc. The successful treatment of the changes (flu, acute bout of congestive heart failure, etc.) will usually result in a return of the person's functioning level to its original state (the level before the onset of that treatable condition).

Should a mentally impaired client experience the flu (upper respiratory infection or diarrhea) the caregiver will likely see a significant decrease in the client's ability, an increase in confusion and possible behavioral response. Anyone experiencing the flu will suffer lethargy or loss of energy and mental sluggishness. Our ability to perform tasks is impaired until the flu is cured. The same is true for those with dementia. When they suffer the flu the related lethargy and mental sluggishness will result in a decrease in cognitive ability, endurance and performance. Even though the person is confused, he is able to wash and dress himself in the morning with little difficulty. While experiencing the flu he is unable to wash or dress himself at that time of the day, has little tolerance when being helped, becoming resistive or even aggressive when the caregiver attempts to help him. When he is over the flu he returns back to his normal functioning level and behavioral response – dressing and feeding himself with little support and little difficulty.

When changes in behavior or functioning ability occur, it is easy to attribute it to part of the disease that is causing the dementia. In reality, any changes should initiate a medical assessment, which is the key to ensuring that any further changes in cognitive functioning are not the result of a treatable secondary disease process.

Approach

We will return to the earlier scenario involving approach a dementia client. Imagine:

> You are mentally impaired
> Sitting in your chair./
> At 0845 hours I enter your room
> To take you to the bathroom./
> Standing over you I ask, "Do you have to go to the washroom?"/
> Without any further direction
> I take you by the elbow to assist you to stand.
> You resist, becoming aggressive and defensive./

The mentally impaired experiences a chronic emotional state of anxiety and fear. With the inability to analyze situations and events, all one can do is read the actions and behaviors of others at face value. This makes a person highly prone to eliciting a defensive response to any situation that is not clearly understood. Taking you by the elbow and making you stand without much warning creates a very threatening experience. Being unable to remember who I am or where you are, you cannot determine where I am taking you. My actions as you see them, justifies only one logical response - to become defensive in order to protect yourself.

If the agitation created by this event ended when you left the room, there would be little problem. That is not always the case. Instead it is more common that the heightened level of fear and anxiety will remain. With some clients it can last for hours, with others the rest of the day.

In fact, this heightened fear and anxiety could spill over to other caregivers, situations and other shifts. That one event could affect the success of the entire care team. During that day, even those who normally have little difficulty taking you to the washroom, may now find you difficult to handle.

Once the anxiety level of the mentally impaired is increased, it may take some time for a sense of security to return. During this heightened anxiety there exists a strong suspicious tendency when interpreting the actions of others. Normal tasks and performance levels will be dramatically affected during this period (diagram #3).

Environment

A team of professionals visited a thirty bed unit for the mentally impaired elderly. Initially they found the majority of clients sitting. They saw little wandering and no agitated behavior. After walking about the unit for only ten minutes, talking to staff and amongst themselves, there was a noted increase in wandering and aggressive behavior of the mentally impaired on that unit.

If a stimulus in the environment cannot easily be identified or clarified by the mentally impaired, it increases anxiety.
An increase in anxiety decreases mental functioning, thereby increasing wandering or agitated behavior.

This is an important concept - anyone in contact with the mentally impaired can influence care. Initially when visiting a unit for the mentally impaired elderly, the majority of clients were sitting quietly in the lounge apparently listening to music from the stereo. There was little wandering or aggressive behavior seen anywhere at this time. The maintenance man walked onto the unit carrying an aluminum ladder. He erected the ladder in front of the lounge door and began tearing tile from the ceiling and shouting to another maintenance man down the hall. Within a short time a number of the mentally impaired clients who were in the lounge became restless and some began wandering. Finally the agitated behavior of other clients in the lounge disrupted the music session.

The clients in the lounge did not understand the noise or where it originated. All they knew was that they heard a noise they could not comprehend. This unknown stimulus increased their anxiety, causing some to wander and others to become agitated.

Previous to that incident, many of the clients in the lounge were able to listen to the music. Once the environment intensified their anxiety, the mental functioning of some to concentrate on that task decreased. As a result, a task that normally could be performed was now severely curtailed. (see diagram #3)

Long term care facilities can present significant challenges. Is there a difference in the activity and noise level on your unit at 1000 hours on Sunday morning compared to 1000 hours Monday morning? If your response is "yes," then you have just authenticated the potential effects of an uncontrolled environment.

While assessing one unit, I stood at what was known as the crossroads (a hall to my back, one to my front and one to the left and right). It was 1000 hours on a Monday morning.

- Located in the corner in front of me and to my left was an open lounge.
- In that lounge the TV and the radio were on at the same time.
- Two very confused clients were talking to themselves quite loudly.
- Another client was yelling to be allowed out of the chair.
- At the opposite corner was the nurse's station. The doctor and nurse were talking about orders.
- The phone was ringing.
- Call bells were sounding.
- The door alarm was initiated.
- Behind me coming up the hall was another client being pushed in a wheelchair. It was time for her bath, and it was definite she did not want a bath given the commotion she demonstrated.
- Above me announcements were heard over the PA system.
- In front of me a housekeeper was running the floor polisher.

Imagine the state and functioning ability of the mentally impaired living on that unit at that time. The problem created remained even after the noise level had subsided. In fact, in this situation the effects of the bombarding lasted for hours. The agitation and confusion level of many of the clients was elevated and their ability to function decreased for some time afterwards.

Each of these factors: drugs, other diseases, approach and environment, can dramatically affect the success of any mentally impaired clients to survive in our environment. Some say that there is little that can be done with the mentally impaired. Given what has just been presented, it is easy to reveal the vulnerability of the mentally impaired. As a result, their need for a controlled, supportive environment demonstrates that there is much that can be done. However, it does not end there. There are more, not so obvious issues that can have a significant impact on the lives of the mentally impaired. Let us examine them to some depth.

Chapter Five

Symptoms

The symptoms associated with mental impairment are varied and complex. There are virtually no two mentally impaired clients with the same combination of symptoms, behaviors and degree of loss in functioning ability. This variance emphasizes the importance of assessment. Until the individual's strengths, limitations and vulnerabilities are defined, care direction cannot be accurately determined.

When discussing the following symptoms, specific assessment mechanisms and guidelines on appropriate care practices will also be presented. Further details of specific supportive measures will be expanded in subsequent chapters.

It is important to emphasize that certain liberties have been taken when discussing the symptoms associated with dementia. Descriptions, definitions and scenarios are presented as they directly impact on functioning ability and the subsequent behavioral response. Investigation into more formal definitions and representations of symptoms may be needed to attain a full appreciation of what is caused by the disease.

Judgment

A behavioral definition of the impairment to judgment represents:

A loss in the ability to differentiate extremes –
the differences between right/wrong; good/bad; too much/too little.

A person with impairment in judgment only knows that something has to be done, so he does it. He cannot define limits or determine the consequences of many of his actions. Examples of the behavioral response by many dementia clients includes:

- putting on three pairs of pants and two shirts when picking out her own clothes.
- becoming bizarre in appearance when applying her make-up.
- pouring coffee into his cereal when given his breakfast.

Usually this person is not aware of there being a problem. In fact, it appears that those with an impairment in judgment are often pleased with what they have accomplished. Not being able to identify any limits to their actions, they are unable to identify when anything is wrong, believing they have done the task appropriately. To collaborate this, watch how a female mentally impaired client responds to her attempt at applying make-up. Even though bizarre in her appearance, she acts as though everything is fine.

Constantly correcting this individual is often not effective and may even lead to an aggressive or wandering response. The behavioral response is due to the obvious conflict of our seeing something wrong when the client feels everything is fine. To say to this person, "Look what you have done to your face," creates a state of confusion. When challenged in such a manner, she will invariably become confused by the comment. As far as she is concerned there is nothing wrong with "her face." This confusion intensifies the feeling of being out of control, increases her anxiety level, and will probably result in an intense behavioral response.

To reprimand her for her action, when she is not aware that her action is inappropriate, will have a detrimental effect. Only minutes after the confrontation, she will probably not remember what was said about her make-up (recent memory loss), but will retain the emotions that were stirred from the comment. Consequently, her aggressive or wandering behavior could last for a significant period and negatively impact on all aspects of subsequent care and programming.

In keeping with the mandate of Supportive Therapy, we must compensate for the individual's limitations and maintain her strengths. The more effective approach is to focus on her strengths, not limitations. In this scenario, her strength is obvious - she attempted to put on her make-up even though she has limited functioning ability. This supportive response: "Mary, you put on your make-up today, good for you. You missed a spot on your cheek with some of your blush. Why don't we go into your room and fix that and you'll look just great." will likely result in her returning to her room more willingly, than by confronting her with what she has done poorly.

The most effective supportive measure involves <u>anticipation</u>. Anticipation is the ability to predict a client's behavior. This allows the caregiver to be prepared for the behavior. If this lady has repeatedly applied her make-up (or someone else's) making her appearance bizarre, then chances are that the next time she has her hands on some make-up she will look the same. Anticipation does not solve the problem, it:

- removes the shock.
- prepares one for what might occur.
- sets in place a reaction that is appropriate to the client's limitations.

The most effective means of determining a client's limitation in judgment involves frequent contact and observation. By identifying specific patterns in behavior, one can also identify the supportive measures required. This ongoing assessment becomes the key to successfully caring for the mentally impaired.

- Bizarre appearance in applying make-up requires someone to guide the client through the process, setting the framework for a very appropriate activity program on a daily basis.

- The client who has difficulty combining clothes, will need them laid out on the bed to decrease the choices required.

- The client who has problems with meal times requires the caregiver to guide him in preparing his cereal or coffee.

The behavioral response will not change. It is our responsibility to anticipate what we will encounter and then be supportive in our response.

Orientation

Impairment in orientation will affect a mentally impaired person's ability to relate to time, person, place and/or thing.

a) Time
Time is meaningless to many of those with dementia. The person's loss of recent memory makes it difficult to keep track of the time, day, month or year.

Knowing the time requires a person to be able to remember at least one point of reference - if today is Monday, then tomorrow is Tuesday. However, if a person cannot remember what is just told to him, then that point of reference is gone and time passage is virtually lost. It becomes impossible for the mentally impaired client to keep track of time for the simple fact that it is always changing. The more severe the person's impairment, the more difficulty they have in identifying time. Some will know the day, but not the time of day; others know the month, but not the day; others only the year; and still others, nothing at all.

Being unable to identify time passage makes it difficult to keep track of the simple progression of the day's events. Breakfast, lunch, supper, bedtime, awakening, bathing now have no reference point. This may result in the client being spontaneous in his actions:

- waking in the early hours of the morning.
- insisting it is time for breakfast.
- resisting going to meals.
- saying he just ate.

- not wanting a bath.
- believing he just had one.

An expectation that the client knows the time of day, let alone the day, can result in considerable resistance.

We become the client's "time piece." Clocks may be valuable to some mentally impaired, but the location and number on the unit is critical. The size and where the clock is placed is one of the factors that will determine if it is used. A clock high on the wall, above eye level will never be seen (out of sight is out of mind). One that is small becomes invisible. Modern digital clocks are of little value to many mentally impaired - seeing the time as 1315 hours is meaningless. The clock must be a large faced clock, with large numbers and hands, located at eye level on a wall that makes it visible from any point in the room.

Before any client is encouraged to read and use a clock, she must be assessed to determine if she can relate to one. To some mentally impaired, looking at even a large faced clock at eye level may provide as much information as looking at a blank wall.

Assessment:

> Place a clock in front of the client and ask him to identify specified times.
> Place the hands of the clock at specific times (8, 12 and 5 o'clock) and ask what would happen at those times (breakfast, lunch and supper).

If she is able to read and understand a clock placed in front of her, then she may be able to use one in her room and in the lounge. If she can identify key times of the day - 8 a.m., 12 noon, 5 p.m., 9 p.m., then she can be provided a schedule of <u>her</u> day in large, bold print identifying breakfast, lunch, supper and bedtime. A clock on its own may be of little value; a clock next to an event board can be useful.

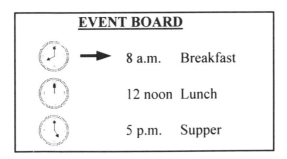

Depending on the client's functioning level, the event board becomes an important reference to identify the next activity. As one event is completed, the arrow is moved down. The clock next to the event board assists the client to determine how long before the next activity. Even if a person is unable to relate to the clock, the sign itself may be of assistance. Spaces are left on the event board after each main function to insert the times of other events for that day (i.e. 10 a.m. - exercises).

By the way, the most successful clock placed in the client's lounge is an old fashioned pendulum chime clock. The intention for this device is not to assist the person in telling time, but to hook "old memories." The chimes will attract the attention of many clients to look at the clock, potentially eliciting many old memories, and providing some interesting conversations.

The importance of constantly reinforcing time to the mentally impaired must be questioned. A popular seminar that I presented was called "Does It Really Matter If Its Tuesday?" At the end of the session, participants would ask, "Does it matter if it is Tuesday to the mentally impaired?" My response was always the same "If the client forgets, you'll remember."

In reality, few low functioning dementia clients are able to relate to complex objects such as clocks, event boards and calendars. That leaves the caregiver as the main vehicle to provide the needed information - the time of the day. Telling the client the day and time does not ensure that she will remember, but ensures the environment in which she lives attempts to compensate for the limitations she experiences.

However, telling the client is based on the client's reaction to the information. If the response is positive or neutral, then it is encouraged that you continue. If the client becomes distressed with the constant reinforcement of time, then the negative consequences indicate that it is inappropriate to continue that practice. Always let the behavioral response of the client direct the actions taken.

b) Place

Impairment in recent memory makes it extremely difficult for a client to remember where he is. The following assessment questions are valuable to determine the degree of disorientation:

> Where are you living now?
> Is this where you work, a hospital, a nursing home or your home?

The inability to respond correctly to the first question initiates the interviewer to ask the second.

The response to these questions provides significant information. Determining where the client believes he is may explain some of the behaviors demonstrated and provide direction on the best course of action to be taken. For example:

- a need to clean, if it is believed to be home.
- an insistence of going home, if it is believed to be work.
- soon to go home, if believed to be a hospital.

It can be understood how believing I am at work or in a hospital initiates an elopement behavior, a need to leave the building for the simple reason - "I don't belong here."

The client's orientation is an important cue for members of the care team. If the client has difficulty remembering where he is, he may also have difficulty relating to staff performing personal care. Imagine the conflict if a client believes the unit on which he lives is his place of employment - no one where he worked ever attempted to drop his pants to take him to the bathroom. It is essential that on each contact caregivers reinforce to this client where he is, who they are and what is about to be done.

Although such a basic approach may be thought common-place, it can be easily overlooked given the number of times it has to be done. Reminding all mentally impaired clients who you are and what you are doing each time you make contact becomes difficult. When you consider the number of mentally impaired clients under your care, the number of times you may make contact with each in that day and the number of days you will be providing care, it is not surprising that it will frequently be neglected.

Behavior care practices need to be specific to the individual's needs. Although reinforcing information is encouraged with all clients, it is *mandatory* on each contact for those identified few who become resistive or aggressive when not told where they are. In that case, all members of the care team (nursing, housekeeping, dietary, administrative, etc.), are expected to always reinforce with these specific clients where they are, who you are and what you are doing on every contact. By limiting the number of clients that need and can relate to this type of reinforcement, we have increased the chances that it will be consistently undertaken by all who are in contact with these individuals.

c) Person
Some mentally impaired clients:

- *can remember faces and names.*
- *some can only remember faces.*
- *others can remember neither.*

A daughter was introducing me to her mother. The mother was mentally impaired and had very poor recent memory retention. Once the introduction was made, the mother said to me, "Who is that standing next to you?" It was the daughter. Mother was incapable of remembering the daughter by name or face. Once the daughter heard mother's question, she became incensed. She said quite indignantly, "Mother, you know who I am. She always does this. She knows who I am when she wants." Wrong! Mother has lost the mental ability to identify most, if not all persons by name or by face. Yet the daughter would not accept her mother's limitation. During our conversation, it was discovered that the daughter spent every visit attempting to have mother address her by name. You can imagine the result of such pressuring on the emotional state of both and how each visit ended.

This expectation that the mentally impaired have the ability to turn memory on and off is deleterious to effective care. It assumes that a person with a destructive brain disorder is able to be selective. That is impossible! Yet some will always argue, "My mother remembers my sister who rarely visits, but she never knows who I am. She is just trying to make me feel guilty for putting her in the nursing home." It is amazing how some consistently ignore the effects of the disease, insisting that mental functioning is still operable.

Some mentally impaired are able to remember faces, but not names. Certain caregivers will enter the room of a specific client and get a very different response than others, such as a smile and a warm greeting. The same is true of family. When the daughter visits, the client may greet her with a hug and a smile. Ask the client who she is and she will probably respond, "I don't know." The client is responding to the familiarity of the face. There is some part of that face she can recall, telling her that she has seen this person before, but she cannot remember where or when. So she responds accordingly.

The ability to remember one face and forget another clearly demonstrates the spotty and random destruction occurring within the brain. There is no conscious selectivity on the part of the mentally impaired. When working with a specific client five days a week for two years, there develops a considerable degree of familiarity on the part of the caregiver. We see that same client each day, and can easily believe the client has the same degree of familiarity. In actual fact, to some clients, each time may be the first time despite how much contact is made with members of the care team.

Assessment:

Does this person work here or live here?

Pointing to another client living within the facility and then to a caregiver and asking the above question of a mentally impaired client will provide considerable information. The ability to know whether the person you are pointing to lives or works here gives a possible indication of the client's response to people approaching him. If incapable of differentiating between staff and other clients, there will be an obvious resistive behavior to being taken to the washroom. Likewise, such a client may mistakenly approach other clients for assistance to the toilet. The delay in finding the right person to take her may be the main cause for her incontinence.

d) Thing

The location of the damage in the brain dictates the information that is lost. The condition of Agnosia identified in a previous chapter demonstrated that a mentally impaired client can lose the ability to:

- identify an object.
- manipulate an object.
- associate a specific word to an object.

It is important to determine which objects in every day use the client is capable of identifying. While interviewing or performing care, simply point to a common object and ask, "What is this?" If she is repeatedly incapable of correctly identifying many objects, then it is important to know what this person can recognize and what she cannot. This information becomes essential for all caregivers in knowing what instructions must be given to her, what should be asked of her and what supports she will require.

To associate a specific word (chair) to the appropriate object requires the person to first form a mental image of that object, then compare that image to something found in the environment that is identical. That is simple enough to demonstrate:

I will provide the following word:

Tree

Now find one! In order to find a tree, you must compare the picture you created in your mind's eye with something identical in the environment. If you were unable to create an image of a tree in your mind, how would you find one?

For some mentally impaired clients, the information required to create the image is lost, making the words meaningless. Some clients, who may not be able to identify an object by name, may still use it and respond appropriately to it if they see the same item (chair). If caregivers are not aware of this limitation with a specific client, it could easily lead to labelling that person as attention seeking or resistive.

Without knowing what a client can identify by word or by sight, it is impossible for the care team to determine how to communicate effectively to any client and be supportive of their limitations during any contact.

Recent Memory

The inability of the mentally impaired to retain recent memory is the main premise for many limitations. Initially, the client may be able to remember up to a month ago. As more and more of the brain is damaged, further memory is lost. At some point the person may be able to recall only specific events that happened years ago.

One of the challenges in working with the mentally impaired is attempting to determine how much memory has been lost. Some are unable to remember much of the past forty years, but can converse in depth about the specific details that occurred on a specific day in the 1940's. This contradiction in ability creates considerable confusion on the part of some family members: "How is it that Dad can remember little things that happened years ago, but cannot remember that I visited yesterday?"

The most basic way to imagine the progression of memory loss in association with the related brain damage is to compare the brain to an onion. Imagine the brain layered like an onion, where recent memory is in the outer layers and older memory closer to the core. As the brain is being destroyed, take a layer away. Of course the brain is not like an "onion," and memory retention is not that simplistic. However, it is an important analogy for two reasons. The first is to demonstrate the progression of memory loss as the disease worsens. The other is to display the permanency. Once a layer of an onion is removed, it cannot be replaced. It is gone. Likewise with the destructive nature of the disease, once memory is lost, it is lost and cannot be put back.

The ability to remember certain aspects of one's life and its history is totally dependent on the location and degree of destruction within the brain. Selective areas of the brain can be destroyed. Whatever information those cells retained will be lost. This re-emphasizes the error made in comparing one mentally impaired client to another. A caregiver believing that both clients in a semi-private room know who she is and what she is doing because one of them has such ability, would have disastrous results.

Assessment:

> How old are you?
> What is your spouse's name?
> How many children do you have?
> What are their ages?
> I will give you three words - house, orange and dog.
> I would like you to remember them (in 5 minutes ask what
> those words were).
> My name is _____ (in 5 minutes ask if he knows your name).

Each of these questions is an opportunity to determine the degree of memory loss experienced. The inability to recall the interviewer's name or three simple words is a good indication of the client's difficulty with recent memory. This person would probably demonstrate a significant problem in following instructions, requiring caregivers to repeat to him what they want done, rather than expecting him to remember the sequence in total.

The challenge is to know what the person can remember. One of the most effective assessment strategies of supportive therapy is to personify: "to get inside that person's mind." Personification is an attempt to know what the person can remember in order to understand his behavior and adjust interventions and approach appropriately.

Some may believe that such a feat is impossible or useless. On the contrary, personification is one of the key skills in achieving empathy, the ability to place ourselves inside the mind of the person under our care. I do not know what it is like to have cancer, be dying or be severely depressed, but through increased contact with those in these states, the opportunity to intuitively understand that person's frame of reference increases. That understanding can be encountered when working with the mentally impaired elderly as well.

One mentally impaired client, when asked the year, would always place his answers around the "1950's." Caregivers and family found that he was continually obsessed about money:

- always telling staff he didn't have enough money.
- trying to pay staff as soon as they completed a task.
- never letting his wallet out of his sight.
- talking about going to the "poor house."

To the care team, this behavior had little meaning until they talked with the client's daughter. From his daughter, caregivers learned that in the late 1950's this client owned and operated his own business. Due to financial difficulty, his business went bankrupt, leaving him unemployed. During that time he was constantly fearful of the family's financial survival. It is not always as obvious as in this case, but if you can identify where the client is in time, you may understand the behaviors he is presenting.

One very important question that must be asked of family in order to assist in understanding where that mentally impaired client may be locked in time is:

What significant events stand out for you
about your mom/dad's life?

Memory is selective. We do not remember every minute of our lives. Instead, we remember things that have strong emotions associated with them, whether positive or negative.

The mentally impaired are virtually in a time warp and function through what can be called *fragmented memory retention*. They interpret events, people and situations based on their place in time and by only limited pieces of that memory. Let me demonstrate.

A mentally impaired client may only be receptive to certain caregivers providing care and resistive to others. The reason may be quite simple. The caregivers she cooperates with wear glasses, and those she fights do not. In this case, she can remember someone in her past that she was fond of who wore glasses. When she sees someone now wearing glasses, it provides familiarity and in turn decreases her anxious state.

We have just demonstrated an important aspect in understanding certain behaviors of the mentally impaired:

To the mentally impaired,
their world is very real
and they respond accordingly.

A gentleman (94 years old) and his wife (87) were living in a long term care facility. The husband was well, both physically and mentally, living on the independent wing of the facility. The wife suffered from Alzheimer's disease, was very impaired and lived on one of the nursing units. I was asked to counsel the husband who was having great difficulty handling his relationship with his wife.

He stated, "When I walk into my wife's room and she sees me, she tries to hit me, bite me and sometimes spit at me. When she sees my son, she calls him by my name. When she sees my daughter, she calls her by her mother's name." The goal again in Supportive Therapy is to attempt to understand the world of the individual under your care - to personify. This method of getting inside that person's mind allows one to speculate what that person sees and experiences. The husband was asked for a recent picture of his son. He produced a picture of a 64 year old man that was the spitting image of his father. When the wife was assessed, it became obvious that her thought process was fragmented and disjointed, but everything she discussed placed her around the age of fifty.

Imagine her situation. She is sitting in her room. In her mind she is in her fifties, and in walks her 64 year old son. To her, he looks just like her husband. In walks her 67 year old daughter, who possibly looks like her mother. She has it straight. She is in her fifties, her son is her husband and her daughter is her mother. Then, in walks her 94 year old husband. Who does he look like? Like her husband only older. Anyone can see the resemblance between the father and his son. Who does he say he is? Her husband. Now she becomes confused. She feels further out of control, her anxiety is elevated and she becomes aggressive when she sees him.

The husband was advised not to stress that he was her husband, but to visit more as a friend to see if the visits could be less stressful. He made another choice - not to visit at all. He could no longer tolerate the aggressive outbursts of his wife and believed that he was making her situation worse. His response, "I have been married to that lady nearly seventy years. I can't treat her only as a friend. It is better not to visit." He defined well the dilemma and pressures experienced by family.

This fragmented memory retention can also work in the positive. On one unit, the majority of caregivers had difficulty getting a mentally impaired client to take a bath. When the case was reviewed it was found that one staff member (Rose) had relative ease in completing the task. To this client, Rose was a long lost friend. The client would do anything for her. There was something about Rose, her hair style, color, facial features or body shape that hooked into the client's past memory. This client was back at that time in her memory process and therefore was willing to allow Rose to perform any care.

This emphasizes a very significant point in the care routine of that unit. It was asked why this client's bath day was restricted to Tuesday only. To have the routine so restrictive required whoever was on duty that day to battle through the bath. Instead, this client's bath should have been scheduled on "Rose's day," being completed only when that specific staff member was on duty, regardless of which day it was. This ensured that the care process was both supportive to the client and the caregivers required to do the care. This demonstrates an important aspect of programming:

The care team must be flexible enough
to adapt to the memory process
that is occurring
and utilize the resources they have available to them.

An important functional assessment question to ask the care team is:

Who has less of a problem,
who has no problem with this client?

The answer to that question will identify the caregiver with the greatest ability to perform intimate tasks or to defuse any behavioral challenge experienced (a major assessment in behavior care practices discussed later).

Affect

Affect refers to emotion. One of the most common emotional states of mentally impaired clients is a <u>flat affect</u> - little or no emotional expression. This person seems to have few highs and few lows, rarely seen to be laughing or crying. He sits expressionless, whether alone or involved with others.

One daughter said, "My father hates me!" She was asked how she knew that. She responded, "I admitted my father to the nursing home when he became too much to handle. Every time I visit, he refuses to smile no matter what I do." That assessment was wrong. It was not that he refused to smile; it was that he could not smile. For this individual, the area of the brain that controls emotional expression was probably severely damaged. The person with flat affect has lost the ability for *spontaneous emotional expression*. That means he cannot take the feelings he is having on the inside and express them non-verbally through a smile, facial expression or eye movements. It is important for family to be made aware that their Dad's lack of expression is not an indication that he has no feeling for them, but only an indication that he is limited in his ability to express it.

In fact, some caregivers will say, "There is no use bringing him to any activities, he never seems to enjoy them." The question must be asked, "When he attends an activity does he participate or observe?" If the answer is "yes" to either, then keep taking him to the activity. Subjectifying this limitation or implying a hidden meaning to his actions can be limiting.

A person with a flat affect will rarely become aggressive. Not only may he be unable to express happy or pleasant emotions, but angry ones as well. There are limitations to this. For some experiencing a flat affect, a response may be elicited at certain times. The person rarely smiles, but if you place your face in front of his, smile or laugh in his direct view, he may respond with a smile in return. That smile will be quickly lost when you withdraw. Likewise, pull this person out of a chair, or speak in a loud and aggressive manner to him and you may get a brief aggressive response that is soon lost. This demonstrates that for some, if the stimulus is intense enough, you may be able to elicit a response from whatever remaining cells in that part of the brain are still intact and functioning.

The other and more difficult emotional change that may occur with the mental impairment is volatile affect. This is the client who is sitting quietly and for no apparent reason becomes aggressive. This aggression may last for twenty minutes or twenty seconds, and for no apparent reason it stops. Emotional control in this state is restricted due to the specific damage within the brain. Volatile affect can occur when cells within the area of the brain that control emotional expression have been damaged, but not destroyed. When damaged, they alter their functioning ability.

This situation can be compared to that of a person who suffers from epilepsy. This is not to say that the interaction is the same, but if you understand epilepsy, you will better understand what is happening to the mentally impaired client who is volatile. An epileptic usually experiences some alteration to specific brain tissue. Under the right circumstances, those altered cells within that specific area become excited, stimulating the brain and causing a convulsion or seizure. Similarly, if cells that control emotional expression within the brain of the mentally impaired are damaged but not destroyed, these cells could fire off, stimulating the area of the brain that controls emotional expression, causing an aggressive outburst. The person can be said to virtually experience an "emotional seizure."

The cue to volatile affect is often a simple fact: this behavior does not usually demonstrate any pattern (time or event) - it is often spontaneous in nature. When these outbursts occur, this individual must not be pushed to be involved in any activities, whether bathing, eating or dressing, etc. Instead, he should be placed in a safe environment, away from any stimulus until it runs its course.

It is important to note that this behavior will stop eventually. The person will revert from volatile affect to flat affect as the cells in the brain controlling emotional expression are destroyed. This is a further example of the progressive nature of this disease.

Analytical Ability or Processing

In behavioural care, loss of analytical ability refers to impairment of problem solving ability resulting in difficulty with sequential thought. Knowing that completing any task involves a series of sequential steps, this limitation will result in even the simplest of tasks becoming a series of problems.

If a client is instructed, "Please go to your room" the problems presented are immediate. Which door do you take to get into the hallway? Once you decide on a specific door then it is not only which direction you go - forward, left or right, but also where did you "come from." The mentally impaired who have difficulty with analytical ability, or sequential thought, will have problems keeping their thoughts in order. Hence, every task may present itself as a series of problems. Problem solving involves abstract thinking, a significant limitation faced by many of those who are mentally impaired.

In fact, limitations in problem solving ability can be so impaired in some that it even affects their wandering ability. When such an individual encounters an obstacle (a secured door or a wall), it creates a major problem that this person may be incapable of solving. On encountering an obstacle in the wandering path, this client will still seem to attempt to go forward. Standing in front of the wall or door, the client ends up walking in one place and will remain there until someone assists him to turn around and go in another direction.

The problem encountered when standing in front of the door or wall is as follows: "I can't go forward. I don't remember where I have come from, or where I am going. Now what do I do, where do I go and how do I get there, turn left, right?" The person is virtually stuck.

It is not uncommon to find, in some instances, a unique relationship developing between this wanderer and another mentally impaired person on the unit who also wanders. The pair seems to always walk together. When one hits the blockade and is stuck, the other, almost on cue, takes her by the shoulders, manually turns her and then they continue down the hall. Talk about being supportive.

Limitations in analytical ability indicate the importance of supportive programming in two areas.

> 1) An environment that communicates to the mentally
> impaired rather than requiring them to function by
> memory only.

> 2) Brief, one step instructions for even the simplest task.

Each of these areas will be expanded further in subsequent chapters.

Progressive Aphasia

This limitation varies from the ability to find specific words to the point where the person is non-communicative. Often a person lacking the "right" word will substitute it with another word or phrase called "word replacement".

You have encountered in your care a client who will say "change my pants." When you examine the gentleman, you find he has not been incontinent. Over time you begin to learn that when he says "change my pants," he means take him to the washroom, or you will have to change his pants. He has lost the ability to express what he is feeling, a need to go to the bathroom; or he has lost the ability to say or recall the word bathroom, so he replaces it with the next best thing ,"change my pants," to communicate his needs.

Learning a person's vocabulary is important. A female client who has lost the ability to say her husband's name, or simply the word husband, may develop her own specific way to communicate. She approaches you and says, "Where is my brother?" Her brother may have just visited an hour before and when you tell her this, her response will be, "Not my brother, my brother." She now uses one word to convey two meanings.

The only way to determine a person's language is by conversing with him. When speaking with a mentally impaired individual it is important to consciously be aware of any patterns that are demonstrated. In this case identifying the number of times the person replaces or exchanges one word for another.

This same approach is significant for caregivers performing care. Identifying patterns where a client constantly refers to "the rag" instead of the towel or "the scoop" instead of a spoon, etc. is the key. You can imagine the elevation in anxiety experienced when the client believes she is saying what she wants, but no one seems to understand her and she has no other way of expressing herself. Once the care team are is familiar with the person's language pattern, they have gained a significant asset in supporting this individual during any activity - understanding what she wants even though the words used have very different meanings.

Progressive Apraxia

This refers to the inability to perform purposeful activity due to a loss of coordination and muscle control. This symptom results in a loss of hand-eye and body coordination, as well as fine muscle movements. With this limitation the individual loses the ability to manipulate objects, even though muscle control seems to be intact in every other way. Progressive apraxia can be mapped over the course of the disease. Initially the person will feed herself with a fork and knife, then she will only use her fork, then only a spoon, then only her fingers and finally stop feeding herself completely. This demonstrates the progressive loss and subsequent supports required. Should the caregiver not be cognisant of the impact of this symptom, the client can be inadvertently pressured to perform at a level beyond their ability. Continually placing a spoon in the person's hand, even though when left alone she puts it down and uses her fingers to eat, is a total disregard of what the client is showing us she cannot do. Serving spaghetti and not providing an alternate finger food may result in significant frustration for the client and/or the caregiver. The key is to remember that the mentally impaired always communicate through their behaviour, to ignore the cues presented is to illicit an undesired behavioral response.

A more serious consequence of this symptom is the loss of the ability to stand or walk safely. The first sign of loss of balance is the need to "glide the wall" when walking down the hall. This is the need to keep his shoulder to the hallway wall or to hold onto to the handrail. Eventually the person will demonstrate difficulty rising from a chair. A client will use a rocking motion to get enough momentum to lift out of the chair, initially re-gaining balance when upright, but eventually becoming unstable and falling. The most common reason that a dementia client is not encouraged to walk on his own is the frequent falls that eventually result. This demonstrates the significance of the environment as a part of programming and behavioral care.

- Placing this client in a chair without armrests will result in chronic wandering or aggressive behavior. When armrests are missing the person cannot relax in the chair without tipping out.

- Clutter in the hall will increase frustration as the person is required to manoeuvre around each object increasing the risk of falling and subsequent aggressive outbursts.

Delusions

Delusions are incorrect beliefs that persist despite all other evidence to the contrary. However, many of these beliefs may have a sound basis for the mentally impaired. Such a client identifies a caregiver or another client as a person who steals or hurts them or can't be trusted, even though that person has done nothing to merit such an accusation. In fact, the anxiety state and memory loss of the mentally impaired may initiate from them a tendency to read things at face value. Seeing a specific nurse handling another client leads to a belief that she may be hurting her and can't be trusted. Remember that to certain mentally impaired clients, this is not a long term care facility and we are not caregivers. Instead it may be work or a bus depot: "What is that young woman doing taking that old lady by the arm? She has no right doing that." An assessment of the situation based on the client's perception.

Delusions may be based on past events. Knowing the mentally impaired maintain past memory, a client's accusation may be a misidentification of the stimulus received. He now sees in another person a characteristic, manner, expression or appearance that reminds him of someone in his past with whom he had a negative experience. That client now associates that experience with this individual and responds accordingly.

The potential delusional effects that can be encountered by the mentally impaired were demonstrated well when assessing a dementia unit in a long term care facility. When I walked onto that unit a confused and disoriented resident looked at me and yelled, "Be careful of that Bugger. He's the one, he can't be trusted. Bugger, Bugger, Bugger, Bugger!" Something of my appearance clicked with this lady to initiate that response, for reasons known only to her. Possibly she has a mistrust of someone with a beard, or I resemble someone she had a bad experience with in her past. In either situation there is little that could be done to correct her behavior towards me. In this instance it was just a matter of time. The more I visited the unit, avoiding making direct contact with her, smiling if I met her in the hall (regardless of her salutation of "Bugger, Bugger . . ."), the less she became threatened. There is no question that had I been required to care for her, there would have been tense moments. In this situation the best approach would be to have someone else complete her care.

Simple things like losing objects and believing you know where they are or should be, or where you saw them last, makes you wonder who is playing games on you when you cannot find them in that location. Losing track of time and the loss of recent memory contributes to the fact that where you saw them last and where they actually were, are not necessarily the same place. You saw them there months ago, but to you that was yesterday. The subsequent response will undoubtedly be, "Who stole them?"

The actions of others become a significant stimulus to initiate suspicious behavior. Hearing others talking, but not being able to hear what they are saying, becomes fertile ground to believe they are talking about you. Encountering another client who is aggressive, or loud and boisterous, can be interpreted as a person who is out to get you.

Remembering that many mentally impaired clients will interpret actions and stimuli at their face value, and that interpretation is based on their existing mental frame of reference, makes it understandable why delusions and suspicious behavior exist.

Hallucinations/Illusions

There is the belief that the mentally impaired frequently hallucinate. In reality, hallucinations may not be as common as once thought. To hallucinate is to see something that is not there. This can occur as a possible symptom due to specific damage within the brain. There is always the potential of a biological cause for most behaviors. It is well known that many drugs can create such a side effect. However, the more common experience may be <u>illusions</u> rather than hallucinations.

An illusion is a misinterpretation of what is seen, heard or experienced. This is a response to the concepts discussed earlier, 'if the stimulus is not intense enough, then it will be missed (not seen or heard) or *misinterpreted.*' If what the person is experiencing is not intense enough, then the client can only relate to it based on what he believes it is. Many examples demonstrate this well.

- The client who bends down frequently to clean the dirt off the floor. Even though staff can see no dirt and attempt to correct her, she is adamant it is dirty. What this person may be seeing is the patterns in the tile or often the numbers of a shuffle board game painted on the hallway floor.

- One gentleman each evening at dusk would call the staff to look out his window at the kids playing in the yard. When staff looked out all they could see were small evergreen trees scattered throughout the yard. To this man, those trees appeared as small children playing in the yard.

- Another lady insisted that her daughter was in the hallway, on the other side of a secured door. In fact, what this client heard was the voices of female staff walking down the hall and past the door. She interpreted these voices as her daughter talking to someone. This was perfectly logical given her frame of reference. Due to her memory impairment she believed that she was living at home with her daughter. It made perfect sense that one of the female voices she heard on the other side of the door had to be her daughter's. A very accurate analysis given the cueing experienced.

The challenge is in understanding what it is that the mentally impaired see or hear, and how they interpret it within their reality. The ability to personify, learning first where that person may be locked in time, and then scanning the environment around him to identifying the possible triggers that may be creating the response is key to interpreting this type of behaviour. Once defined, then the ability to be supportive is increased allowing for appropriate supportive measures to be implemented specific to that person's needs.

Decreased Attention Span

Depending on the severity of recent memory loss, concentration is easily impaired. Recent memory loss can be so intense that when an individual leaves her room, planning to go to the dining room, she forgets where she is going once she walks through her bedroom door. Such an individual would have considerable difficulty performing any tasks that have multiple steps, following any instructions, or even maintaining a conversation.

To perform a task requires an individual to remember a sequence of events - what was just completed and what needs to be completed now. The person begins to eat, becomes distracted and then leaves the table, forgetting about the food that was left behind. Similarly, when asked to perform an activity, instructions are lost, concentrating on step one, the person forgets step two and loses track of the entire process, until the sequence is easily abandoned. At that point it is easy to be distracted and wander away from the activity.

That explains why many mentally impaired clients have difficulty carrying on a conversation for any length of time. Conversation requires considerable concentration. In order to successfully maintain a conversation, the client must be able to remember what was just said to determine an appropriate response. Poor recent memory easily knocks that sequence off balance. The person finds it difficult to keep track of the topic and rambles from one issue to another.

Mimicking Behavior

Certain mentally impaired clients will mimic almost any behavior - wandering, restlessness, agitation, etc. We established earlier that if the stimulus is not intense enough, it will be missed or misinterpreted. For some mentally impaired the opposite is also true:

If the stimulus is too intense
they cannot help but respond.

Within minutes of care team sitting at a dining room table for a care conference, who is sitting around them? The stimulus is too intense. Clients wandering about see a group of people sitting at a table. The need to investigate in order to understand the environment elicits a response that might be compared to - "I wonder what they are doing? I will find out." Then that person sits with the group.

Even restless behavior can be contagious. One female client on a unit for the mentally impaired was a full time caregiver. Not a nurse or social worker, but throughout her life she would always search for those in need - disabled, mentally handicapped, financially impoverished - and help them, whether they wanted her help or not. Now she was on a unit with thirty mentally impaired older people. To her this must have seemed like "manna from heaven." At mealtime, like many caregivers, she would never think of sitting down and eating before all the rest at her table were settled and eating. Dietary staff would place her plate in front of her, but she would stand up and go to the client sitting next to her, saying, "How are you dear? You have too much of this, let's give some to him. He has too much of this, let's give . . ." She would proceed to take food from one client and give it to another. Eventually every client at that table was into everyone else's food. They began mimicking her restless behavior.

Some mentally impaired will mimic agitation. On another unit there was a female client in her nineties. Whenever she was placed at a table she would pound on it and yell at the top of her lungs, "LUNCH, LUNCH, LUNCH, LUNCH, . . ." regardless of which meal was being served. The effect her screaming and pounding had on other clients was to create a scenario that resembled a prison riot. Clients sitting in the dining room at her table who could normally concentrate on their meal and were fairly quiet, began screaming and hitting the top of the table, mimicking her behavior.

The concept of individualized care is not something that is desirable only for those with dementia, it is also essential to address the behavioral demands that are easily present. The most basic of concepts to emphasize the challenges that face the caregiver are:

- the symptoms of mental impairment are many and complex.
- no two dementia clients experience the same combination and severity of symptoms.
- the progressive nature of the disease means that symptoms are always changing.
- there is little universality in the approach and care concepts implemented.

This individuality requires that programming be determined not by the person's diagnosis, but by his strengths, limitations and vulnerabilities. To dance effectively with the client is to "chase the disease down" - to determine what the client requires at any given time as the disease progresses.

Before we can examine specific supportive measures, it is important to relate these symptoms to the day-to-day encounters of the caregiver. It is one thing to talk about what the person can or cannot do; it is another to identify how his actions affect care and the ability of the care team to be supportive.

Chapter Six

Behavioral Response

All assessment, analysis, programming and environmental supportive measures created within Supportive Therapy are directly related to the specific concepts that initiate a behavioral response by a dementia client. These concepts:

- demonstrate the variation in behavior and functioning when the dementia client is exposed to changes within their environment.
- define the causative factors causing the behavioral response.
- provide the rationale for the assessment tools and supportive measures used.

Before formal behavior care practices can be presented, it is necessary to expanded these concepts as they relate to the day-to-day experiences of the mentally impaired. The concepts discussed within this chapter include:

- Change Response
- Lack of Familiarity
- Bombarding
- Decreased Contact
- Change in Approach
- Change in Energy
- Change in Lighting

- Staff Change
- Loss of Familiarity
- False Cueing
- Noise
- External Factors
- Pre-morbid Personality
- Depression

We will examine the impact of these concepts on functioning ability and behavior as they relate to the client's ability to perform simple tasks and the changes witnessed over a 24 hour period.

Performing Tasks

Imagine:

> You are caring for a mentally impaired client.
> You sit her at her bedside/
> Give her a basin, a towel and a face cloth
> She washes her face and hands./
>
> It is Tuesday morning./
> You take that same client for her weekly bath.
> You place her in the tub
> Hand her the face cloth
> She just stares at it./

There are many factors that come into play to possibly create this change in functioning ability (being able to wash one's face and hands in one location and not in another), they are:

1) Change Response
With the mentally impaired elderly, any task that is changed slightly may become a new task. Adjusting to change requires a very complex, abstract cognitive process called problem solving. The client must:

- compare the "new" situation with the "old" one.
- identify what part of it has changed.
- decide what must be done differently now.

To many mentally impaired clients this level of cognitive functioning is impossible. The Change Response dictates that the slightest change in the environment or what is being asked, may result in any task appearing as though it was new.

This limitation can be encountered when a client experiences a simple change in location or position - from sitting at the side of the bed with a face cloth and basin to sitting in a tub with just a face cloth. While in the tub how do you get the face cloth wet and where do you wring it out? Placing it in the water at your lap is much different from placing it in the water in a basin.

2) Lack of Familiarity

We have established that changing a mentally impaired client from the familiar to the unfamiliar increases anxiety. When anxiety increases mental functioning ability decreases.

A task a client may complete in one setting, may be lost in another simply due to his/her emotional state. Moving a client from her room, where she has considerable familiarity, to a tub room she only encounters once a week will have that effect. Being in the tub room last week, does not mean she remembers where she is now. She can easily be distracted by the noise, lighting, equipment, and staff movements of this new environment. Asking her to use the face cloth in this new environment causes considerable difficulty. She cannot concentrate on the task when distracted by the new stimulus.

3) Bombarding

> What would happen to a mentally impaired client who is asked to do <u>ten</u> things at once?

Usually that client is unable to perform any of them successfully. Asking a client to wash her face and hands at her bedside requires her to concentrate only on one task. Asking her to do the same task in the tub is very different. In the tub room she is exposed to a number of things all at once. To demonstrate the pressures, have that mentally impaired client be you.

Imagine:

I take you to the tub room./
Are you in the same building?/
You are afraid I may leave you there alone.
I undress you completely.
Get you in the tub.
Is the water too hot or too cold?
You have to wash your face.
Your arms
Your neck
Chest
Torso
Legs
Feet
Hair
Get you out of the tub.
Get you dried.
Dressed.
Leave./

All in ten minutes!

Bombarding is asking an individual to perform multiple, separate tasks in a short duration. This often results in the person being unable to perform any successfully.

Imagine what a mentally impaired client goes through. Each task requires considerable thought and concentration. As the client is working to complete one task, it becomes impossible to analyze quickly enough what has to be done to be prepared for the second one. Each bit of information and expectation only further complicates what has to be completed. This saturation of stimuli intensifies anxiety, limiting cognitive ability even further.

Caregivers who can relate to this change in functioning adjust their demands on the client accordingly - assisting the client where needed without criticism. Those who view the change subjectively, usually believe that if this client can perform in a certain manner in one location, then she should <u>always</u> be able to perform in the same manner regardless of place or time. Any alteration in performance is then interpreted as a conscious decision by the client to be resistive or attention seeking.

When a client has right sided paralysis, caregivers would not consider pressuring that person to pick up his fork with his right hand. It is beyond his functioning ability. Likewise:

The mentally impaired client cannot be expected
to perform beyond their functioning abilities.

Given the effects described above, the client has been placed in a situation that is beyond her ability to cope. Pressuring her to wash her face and hands on her own while in the tub will only result in increasing her frustration and anxiety level. This will undoubtedly lead to an aggressive response.

It is not suggested that we take over every task for each mentally impaired client who shows difficulty in functioning. Rather, this emphasizes that a universal approach in dealing with this clientele is not effective.

Certain impaired clients will only perform a task with strong encouragement. To constantly "take over" or rescue such an individual defeats the goal of Supportive Therapy - identifying the person's strengths and maintaining them. The main focus in approach is flexibility. Success in working with any client is based on knowing that client's abilities and limitations. That requires time and successful sharing among the care team to ensure a consistent approach and realistic goals.

Those who have worked with the mentally impaired for any length of time (either professional or family caregivers) have discovered the best approach is one of trial and error. This is not a haphazard approach in dealing with the mentally impaired. It is a successful assessment strategy to determine the most appropriate programming. The process of using trial and error involves attempting something, observing the person's response and assisting when it becomes obvious the person's anxiety level is increasing. It is essential then that all involved in the care of this client maintain the approach or programming that is discovered to be effective.

24 Hour Effect

The 24 Hour Effect represents the differences experienced by a dementia client over a 24 hour period, including: decreased contact, change in approach, change in energy, change in lighting, staff change, loss of familiarity, false cueing and noise.

These differences can so dramatically alter the behavior and/or function ability of a dementia client that they give the impression the person has three different "personalities" and functioning levels over a three shift period. Let us examine these changes and the impact they have on each shift within a health care facility (acute and long term care). Community support staff and family caregivers will encounter many of these similar dynamics in the home setting.

Day Shift to Evening Shift

1) Decreased Contact
In the majority of health care facilities, there are more staff on duty during the day shift than the afternoon shift - more nursing staff, plus housekeeping, recreation, dietary, volunteers and management staff. During the afternoon shift, probably only nursing staff are on duty at a reduced number compared to the day shift.

The higher ratio of staff to clients on the day shift increases the frequency of staff/client contact. Given the principal concept that a dementia client will become more confused the longer the person is left alone, frequent contact increases the opportunity for a client to be more oriented to his surroundings, responding to requests made of him. Conversely, during the afternoon shift a client may be left alone for longer periods, increasing his disorientation, making him less cooperative.

These dynamics can be demonstrated with the following example. At 1000 hours, a housekeeper is in a client's bedroom conversing with the client as she cleans. At 1015 hours the nurse enters the room to take the client to the bathroom. The earlier contact with the housekeeper increases the possibility that the client will maintain a better awareness of those around him and be able to respond more appropriately to the nurse when asked to move from one location to another.

On the afternoon shift the situation changes. A client may have contact with a caregiver at 1730 hours and not again until 1900 hours or later. During that period alone, the client's orientation to his surroundings will probably decrease (the longer a mentally impaired client is left alone, the more confused he will become). When a caregiver attempts to take him to the washroom at 1900 hours, he may become less cooperative, not knowing immediately where he is and who this person may be. A significant change in functioning is shown over a 12 hour period.

2) Change in Approach

If on the day shift (or any other shift), caregivers are positive in their approach - giving the client time to perform tasks, adjusting tasks as needed, being supportive and flexible in that person's routine - the client's anxiety will be low, allowing the client to perform at his maximum level. If during the next shift, those on duty are more structured and task oriented - performing care in a hurried, somewhat mechanical manner - anxiety will be increased. This change in approach will result in a client no longer being able to successfully perform tasks completed easily on the previous shift.

3) Change in Energy

> Imagine what it would be like to do a mentally taxing task for twelve hours straight without a break.

The effect is similar to what a mentally impaired client experiences in a health care facility from 0700 to 1900 hours each day. Every task, stimulus, noise, every person, has to be continually analyzed. By the twelfth hour she would be exhausted. Tasks easily performed earlier in the day, become more and more difficult as her physical and mental energy is depleted. As she becomes tired, her tolerance level deteriorates, decreasing her ability to concentrate and perform the task effectively.

4) Change in Lighting
Many mentally impaired clients develop "anchors" in the environment - using a specific object in a room to help identify their location, rather than trying to remember the room itself.

Probably the best anchor utilized by many mentally impaired clients is a comforter or personal bedspread on their bed. As long as the client can see his bedspread, he knows it is his room. To demonstrate how significant the bedspread is, just remove it from that client's bed and place it on someone else's. Now that becomes that person's room. The room is found by locating the anchor or object.

Imagine:

> I am a mentally impaired client.
> Easily disoriented./
> To locate where I eat
> I wander
> Until I find "my table."/
> A long rectangular table in a corner.
> I normally sit on the chair at the end./
>
> At breakfast and lunch
> I have no trouble finding "my table."/
> I walk directly into the dining room unassisted./
> At supper it is different./
> I wander the halls
> Requiring the staff to take me to the dining room for my
> meal./

During the day, there are often two sources of lighting in every room - direct and indirect. Direct lighting is from the room lighting above, and indirect lighting from the daylight through the windows. Usually both sources of light during the day place the shadows below the objects in the room making objects clearly visible to the mentally impaired.

During the evening the light changes. With the sun setting, the main source of lighting is often only from the ceiling. If that lighting is poor or directional lighting (narrow or concentrated beam), it creates shadows. Shadows are an obscure stimuli (if the stimulus is not intense enough it will be missed or misinterpreted). The table now has a shadow along one side that makes it appear more square in shape than rectangular. As a result, the client may find "his table" in the dining room at breakfast and lunch (minimal shadows), but wanders aimlessly about the unit looking for his table, due to the distortion effect created by the shadows. The distortions from day to evening created by different lighting is called the "sundown syndrome."

The combined effects of all of these changes - changes in staff numbers, staff approach, energy and lighting - may have a significant effect on a client's functioning level from day shift to afternoons.

> You bring me my breakfast tray.
> I feed myself./
> You bring me my lunch tray.
> I feed myself./
> You bring me my supper tray.
> I stare at it./

Those who understand the mentally impaired and how they are affected by different events, will assist the client during supper, realizing his needs change at certain times of the day.

Caregivers who lack this sensitivity may view the client's inability to feed himself supper only as a conscious decision to be difficult or gain attention. Any pressure for the client to perform will result in any possible behavioral response.

Evening Shift to Night Shift

A client wakes at 0200 hours, what does she experience?

1) Staff Change
This is the most devious staff change of them all. When she went to bed at 2100 hours, one group of caregivers were on duty. When she wakes at 0200 hours, there is a different group. She did not see the caregivers change. Her inability to relate to what happened can cause further disorientation, increasing her anxiety level.

2) Loss of Familiarity
We have already established that many mentally impaired clients identify anchors in their environment - one cue that will provide the needed information to tell them where they are. Darkness eliminates all cueing. When a client wakes during the night, she is unable to see the objects within her room that provide familiarity, her disorientation will elevate her fear level, decreasing her functioning ability and/or intensifying her common behavioral response.

3) False Cueing
During the night there are a number of cues that may be difficult for a mentally impaired client to decipher. Waking at two in the morning and believing one is at home does not explain:

- why there are bars on the sides of the bed that won't let her get out of bed (bed side rails are up).
- who that person is in the next bed (roommate).
- who is walking in with a flashlight (staff making rounds).

The inability to clearly define these cues results in considerable fear over what one is experiencing.

4) Noise

> Tonight you are home alone.
> The house is empty./
> You go to sleep./
> At 0300 hours you are awakened
> By a sound you have never heard before./
> Go back to sleep./

During the day and evening shift, background noise on the unit muffles anyone calling out from their room. During the night shift it is different. When a mentally impaired client wakes in the middle of the night, the darkness can disorientate her to believe that she is home. If from the next room she hears a male mentally impaired client yelling in response to a caregiver washing him - "LEAVE ME ALONE. HELP. THEY ARE TRYING TO KILL ME!" The associated fear to such a stimuli would be intense.

All noises in the dark are amplified and more confusing. Caregivers walking by, people talking in the hall, equipment being moved up and down the corridor, call bells sounding, etc. all have the potential to increase the confusion and fear level of any dementia client, inadvertently changing behavior and/or functioning ability.

5) External Factors

External factors involve those things that can increase confusion further. If an individual is taking sleeping medication, that medication has it's greatest impact during the early hours of the morning. If she awakes during those hours, the effect of the medication will only increase her confusion. Likewise, a client who is wakened by a dream or a nightmare, will not know what is real or imagined. An experience we have all encountered.

Mentally impaired clients who wake early in the morning, experience considerable anxiety and intensified disorientation. Caregivers who relate well to this clientele know the best approach to employ - simply allow the client to get up, take him to the lounge, give him a cup of tea and toast, and talk to him for awhile.

This simple supportive measure provides the client the needed sense of security, allowing him to become more oriented to his surroundings and to the people around him. After a few moments the chances are good that the client will return to bed and sleep the rest of the night, or sleep in the chair in the lounge till morning.

However, caregivers who are task oriented take a different approach. They dictate the "rules" (legitimate or not) that clients are to stay in bed and sleep until 0600 hours. These individuals struggle to keep a client in bed and have him "go back to sleep." This only causes the client to become agitated, further restricting his ability to sleep. Unfortunately, the consequences of such an approach is not restricted to the night shift. This client's agitation can easily spill over to the day shift and possibly even the next evening shift, resulting in all caregivers having difficulty performing care.

The difference is dramatic - pressure a mentally impaired client to stay in bed and sleep; or allow the client to get up, get dressed, wander a bit and finally sit in a lounge chair and sleep till six. The most successful tactic in approaching the mentally impaired is flexibility. There is no schedule the mentally impaired can maintain other than their own.

Pre-morbid Personality

Many talk about the personality changes experienced by dementia, however the individual's pre-morbid personality plays an even greater role in influencing behavior. Pre-morbid personality represents the personality characteristics the client had before the onset of dementia.

Imagine:

> During my entire life
> My normal tone & manner of speaking

Is loud & aggressive./
In a conflict situation
I only get louder, more aggressive
And interject a few four letter words to emphasize my point./

I am now 78 years old.
I still have the same boisterous manner./
My wife, who has been married to me for over fifty years
Has learned to cope with my volume and behavior
By going "deaf,"
Not listening to the tone or the words used./

I am now 80 years old
Mentally impaired
A client on your unit./
Being under considerable stress and conflict/
How do I talk to everyone around me?

Inadvertently, the client will respond in the same manner as the past.

The dementia client will commonly maintain a ritualistic pattern - walk the same path, sit in the same chair, do the same things, respond in the same way, etc. This ritualistic pattern creates familiarity. Personality characteristics, mannerisms and behavior the client had before the onset of dementia will not only remain but probably intensify as the disease progresses.

In the past when the client was cognitively well, the client's boisterous nature was controlled by his sensitivity to the response of others. The reaction by others, the situation or presence of certain individuals would result in his being more guarded with his language and mannerisms. Now that he is mentally impaired, he can no longer read in others how his behavior and language affects them (their facial expressions or actions). Words in the past he would never say in mixed company, spill out now no matter who is around. The "taboos" have been forgotten due to his loss of inhibition and analytical ability.

The frustration with this client occurs in the varied responses by caregivers to his behavior. Some have no problem performing the necessary care with this type of client, while others are constantly intimidated or at logger heads with him.

The caregivers who handle this situation well probably respond to his loud and boisterous manner in the same way as his wife during their fifty years of marriage - they will go "deaf" to his onslaught, listening to what he is saying, but ignoring the manner in which it is said.

Caregivers who cannot "tune out," may personalize each encounter, believing he "should" be able to control himself and understand that he is upsetting everyone by his language. The belief that his behavior is within his control results in their attempting to subdue him, to make him more cooperative. Unfortunately their pressuring him to change has an opposite effect - it increases his anxiety, causing even more agitated behavior. Some caregivers forget that even if he did quiet down when asked to, in no time he would forget what was asked and return to "his normal behavior" within minutes.

This is not to suggest that the client's behavior should continue unchecked. This person is living in a communal environment where the rights and safety of others must be maintained. Furthermore, when his behavior intensifies it probably signals that something is distressing him.

Without formal assessment tools revealing the cause of the behavior (Care Analysis), defined supportive measures (24 Hour Profile) and a mechanism to communicate those to all caregivers (Care Plan Summary), there will always be conflict on what should be done.

Caregivers who can relate to such a client, will take the first barrage of insults by ignoring it. By being supportive, they can usually calm him down to the point where he will speak more softly and complete the task asked of him.

Other caregivers are only successful in intensifying his behavior, which may result in their requesting a more drastic option to be taken - sedate him to quiet him down.

The results can be dramatic in some settings. Those who work well with this client may return after a few days off to find him sedated in order to control his behavior. They cannot understand why this client is medicated and find that the drug not only quiets him down, but decreases his ability to function at all other tasks as well.

This scenario, demonstrates the challenge the second half of the definition of behavior management can create for some.

The attempt to control the factors that have further complicated the person's life *in order for the person to maintain the original self.*

"Old behavior" is impossible to change. To establish an effective supportive environment for this client, caregivers must be consistent in their expectations.

Depression

Depression is a debilitating disorder. If not recognized it can even incapacitate the ability of a cognitively well individual and decrease his effectiveness. It is believed that 75% of those with dementia experience depression. The mentally impaired may not know what they have lost specifically, but there is a constant feeling that something is missing, hence the depressive response. This is demonstrated well by the associated feelings of anxiety and the constant "looking for something familiar" in order to control their environment.

The common symptoms characteristic of depression are also common symptoms associated with the brain damage caused by Alzheimer's disease and other dementias:

Loss of appetite
Loss of weight
Decrease of energy causing lethargy
Constipation

    Anxiety
    Withdrawal
    Retardation of thought and action
    Feelings of worthlessness
    Apathy to environment and activities of daily living
    And *Confusion.*

This demonstrates the potential impact depression can have to further complicate the situation and decrease mental functioning.

Given the susceptibility to depression, it is worth treating a mentally impaired client with an anti-depressive agent. If there is an apparent mood elevation, then stay with the drug. If there is no change, then discontinue it.

Chapter Seven

The Challenges

There is no cookbook or magic formula when caring for the mentally impaired elderly. Each caregiver must determine on every contact what is needed and how it must be satisfied with every mentally impaired client.

This text has frequently emphasized the limitation of our role. Many times, success in care is not in changing the client's behavior, but the caregiver's reaction to the situation. In reality, caring for the mentally impaired requires a constant demand for assessment, creativity, flexibility, compassion, high energy and more.

Integrated Environment

An integrated environment, mixing cognitively well/physically disabled clients with the mentally impaired on the same unit creates its own challenges.

Imagine:

> You are assigned to eight clients.
> Four are cognitively well, four are mentally impaired./
> You walk into the room of your first cognitively well client.
> Your expectations of this person's performance are high./
> She knows right from wrong.
> She can problem solve.
> When you give her specific instructions
> She can clarify them if she does not understand./
> If she needs anything, she will ask./

You walk into the room of your next client,
Another who is cognitively well./
Again your expectations of her performance are high./

You enter the room of your seventh client.
This person is mentally impaired./
When you pull back the covers in his bed
You find that he is covered in his own feces/
With his hands smearing it about./

The automatic response by some may be, "Mr. Jones get your hands out of there. How many times have you been told?" It becomes difficult to maintain one's objectivity under such circumstances. This scenario needs to be examined from both points of view, first the client's and then the staff's.

Are the mentally impaired aware of being incontinent of urine or involuntary of stool?

Some may not, but a majority appear to be. Depending on the person's cognitive functioning level, if a mentally impaired client is left sitting with her clothing wet for any length of time, she will usually become restless, at times attempting to remove the soiled clothing herself.

This is not to say that the mentally impaired are aware of what they have done, but possibly more aware of there being a problem causing them to feel uncomfortable. Toilet training is the first thing we learn in our maturing years and the last sensation for many to lose.

If early in the morning a mentally impaired client is lying in bed with the side rails up, and he needs to go to the bathroom, what does he do? He does not have the cognitive ability to use the call bell. He does not know that pushing the button summons a person who would take him to the bathroom. All he knows is he has "to go." So he "goes."

What may contribute to the "smearing" of feces in the bed may be simple, most of our clients have been caregivers all of their lives, not care receivers. The majority have had a lifestyle which dictated that when they encountered a "mess" they would clean it up. Now in his bed is a "mess." He either places it in his water jug (the only available receptacle) or cleans it up (result of old behavior). Being mentally impaired, the more he attempts to clean the "mess," the worse it becomes. The point being emphasized is that the person is attempting to function at his maximum ability.

A caregiver walks into the room and sees him smearing the feces about. It is easy to believe that he is "playing with it," not knowing he is trying to help. Some are able to maintain their composure and be objective about the situation, seeing it through the client's perspective. Others have difficulty maintaining objectivity during every problem. As a result, the client is pressured to function as though he is cognitively well, expecting him to know that what he is doing is "wrong." An expectation that is beyond his ability.

Caregivers working on an integrated unit cannot be blamed for the times they lose their objectivity. It is difficult to always remember that the person in front of you is mentally impaired, when most of the morning you have been working with cognitively well, physically disabled clients.

After leaving the last cognitively well client, one's expectations of that person's functioning was high - the person was able to understand what was expected of her, what was right and wrong. Knowing that you are walking into the room of your first mentally impaired client may not be enough to sufficiently change your perspective. The problem is a simple one - this client looks just like all other clients. In other words, he looks normal but is acting inappropriately. It is difficult to adjust one's approach and expectations when you cannot see the limitations in order to judge the direction of care.

The frustrations experienced with a mixed client assignment (cognitively well/physically disabled, and mentally impaired) is that in seconds caregivers must completely adjust their approach and expectations. Not an easy task for even the most skilled caregiver. It is so natural to say something to a mentally impaired client in such a setting, then turn and ask yourself why you said it. You become aware afterwards that he may not understand what you are talking about.

This scenario, which is so frequently encountered on an integrated unit, can be compared to taking a medical unit and psychiatric unit of an acute care hospital and intermixing them. This would result in staff caring for two patients in a semi-private bedroom:

- One patient in the first bed is admitted for a cholecystectomy - removal of her gallbladder.
- The other patient in that room is a full blown psychotic schizophrenic (severe mental disorder, that can present very bizarre behavior) in an acute state.

Would the care team have difficulty performing care?

Absolutely! We have two specialties in long term care - caring for the cognitively well, physically disabled, and caring for the mentally impaired elderly. The concepts of each is different than the other. Yet on an integrated unit there seems to be little sensitivity to the pressures it creates. Perhaps we should examine levels of care assignments in general in our facilities, before expecting too much from the caregivers themselves (see Modular Care).

Reactive

What is frustrating in working with the mentally impaired is that we do not know what they see, hear or feel. An 80 year old mentally impaired client says, "Have you seen my mother? I just saw her going down the hall!" No matter what she is told, she insists she just saw her. The client is locked into past memories, at a time when her mother was alive and part of her life. When she sees someone walk by who has similar features to her mother (same body build, hair style, etc.) it is easy to believe that was her. The client is reactive, responding to things as she sees, hears and feels them.

The world of the mentally impaired is very real. They will interpret what they see, feel and hear based on how it fits into their reality. There are many examples:

A chair leg that squeals as it is dragged across the floor may initiate a client who has lived with a cat all of her life to respond, "Those boys are hurting the cat again."

Hearing her daughter out in the hall, when she really hears staff talking as they walk past the door.

Looking for the "baby" when she in actual fact is hearing another client crying out in another room down the hall.

Seeing someone that resembles a person in their past and calling that person by that long forgotten name.

Angry that the person who is talking to her will not answer her questions, when she is actually overhearing voices from the TV.

Our frustration as caregivers results from our inability to see the world as the client sees it, making it difficult at times to be supportive when we don't know what we are to be supportive of. This only emphasizes the continual need to personify. To get inside that person's head. To always attempt to see the world as the mentally impaired may see it in order to understand their behavior. Effective personification is the result of repeated exposure to that specific individual; determining patterns of behavior to be able to identify what that person may be encountering; knowing this person's history or past; and having effective assessments tools at one's disposal.

Manipulative Behavior

Can the mentally impaired manipulate?

NO! It is cognitively impossible for a mentally impaired client to manipulate. In order to manipulate, one requires two pieces of information - knowing available options and the "cause and effect" relationship of their actions. This can be demonstrated in the following manner.

If you have children, you have potential manipulators. Again, it is not to imply that older adults are like children, but the behavior demonstrated by children clearly demonstrates the skills needed in order to manipulate.

Imagine:

> You are my mother./
> I am 4 years old./
> I approach you in the kitchen,
> "Mom I want to play with you."/
> You respond, "Len, I am busy right now,
> Why don't you go to your room for a bit and play.
> I will be up later to spend some time with you."/

It is remarkable that when a child's immediate needs are denied, anything that can break in the house will probably get broken at that exact moment. This child knows his options.

- One of his options is to return to his room and wait.
- The other is to return to mom and say, "Mom I don't care if you're busy or not, I want to play with you NOW." That would have a specific response.
- The third option is to get mother's attention by doing something that will require her to "come running." This is better termed "pushing mom's buttons."

The decision he makes is at a conscious and well thought-out level.

This child knows "cause and effect." He is aware that he can do things that will make mother run to him when he wants her, like knock a vase off the table. You can see his mind working even before he knocks over the vase. He looks from one side to the other to see if mother will be in "ear shot" of the noise created when it hits the floor. If mother is not around, the vase may very well stay on the table - why waste energy for little gain - if mother can't hear it hit the floor, he won't get the response he wants.

If you are married follow through with this scenario. If you are not, imagine what the responses may be.

Does your spouse know you?

He may not know you the way you may want him to, but does he know when you are hurting emotionally and when to come close? Again it may not be the degree or type of support that you want, but does he respond?

Does he know when you are angry, and to stay away?

Again his response to your anger may not be exactly when and how you want it.

If your answer is no, then you have not looked closely enough at your relationship. You cannot live intimately with someone without gaining a "hand/glove" relationship. Intimate contact every day, each year creates a reflex response neither spouse may be fully aware of. In the years that you are married, subtle cues from one partner to the other are identified and responded to, often at an unconscious level. The manner and degree of response may not be what the other partner expects or wants, but there is usually a response. To understand the subtleties of such a long term relationship, just ask a widow what she lost when she lost her husband. She will usually respond that there are things missing now that she was not even conscious of while he was alive.

You are now 78 years old.
Your spouse is dead.
You are mentally impaired
Living on a long term care unit./

Would caregivers know you as intimately?

How will they know when you are hurting emotionally?

They can never know you to the degree of your spouse. Caregivers will usually read your emotional distress when there is a more obvious cue like *crying*. In realty, you never had to cry for your husband to know that you were hurting. Your husband only had to see the look in your eyes, your expression, or hear a specific tone in your voice to know that there was a problem that required his support.

How will caregivers know when you are angry?

Only when you become *aggressive*. Again you rarely had to show your husband such an intense response. He only had to see the subtle cues - the look in your eye, what you did, to know that you were upset.

Is it possible to teach you now at 78 years old, mentally impaired, living in a long term care facility how to deal with your emotional needs differently? You are left only to respond to your needs at a "gut level." When you are afraid, you call "Mother, mother, mother, . . ." or "Ow, Ow, Ow, . . ." until someone comes to you, talks with you, touches you. Or when you are angry, you bite, spit, kick, until they leave you alone.

The mentally impaired cannot manipulate! They do not have the cognitive ability to problem solve in order to decide what options are available, to resolve what they are experiencing, and have their needs met. Even if told the acceptable options to get a caregiver's attention or to be left alone, a few moments later they will forget those instructions and resume their previous behavior. Likewise, they do not have the insight to determine cause and effect. Such an analytical process is beyond their ability.

This implies a significant aspect of understanding limitations in care. First, a program called behavior modification is probably one of the cruelest things that could be done to a level two mentally impaired client. It is important to differentiate behavior modification from behavior management. The definition of behavior modification is:

> An attempt to modify or change the person in order
> to decrease or eliminate the undesired behavior.

This is rewarding a client when the desired behavior is demonstrated or withholding from the client something of importance when the undesired behavior is presented, i.e. knowing that a client enjoys a cup of coffee and making that as the incentive for the client to stop her behavior. When used with the mentally impaired elderly this is paramount to abuse - intentionally withholding a component of the individual's quality of life to control something beyond her ability.

When a mentally impaired client is told that if she stops calling out for fifteen minutes she will receive a cup of coffee, she may respond "Okay." Just as soon as the caregiver walks out of the room, she will call out again. Her loss of analytical ability means that she may not understand the instructions given to her on the alternate behavior; her poor recent memory retention will mean that she cannot remember what was told to her. Her behavior will not stop by simply giving her alternate instructions.

Likewise, this refutes those caregivers who believe that she can stop calling out if she wants. This lady knows nothing of cause and effect. She has a need and responds accordingly. She does not even know if calling repeatedly will have any results. She just calls until there is a response. Besides, if she does stop calling, how does she get you?

What the mentally impaired must do is respond to their needs - doing what is necessary given the circumstances experienced at that specific time. A very basic human response.

Qualities of a Caregiver

This book has emphasized that successful caring of the mentally impaired is dependent on how caregivers perform that care. Those who are successful possess some very unique qualities. They must be:

> Part Elephant
> Part Duck
> Eyes of a Hawk
> Patience of a Saint
> Rationality of Mr. Spock
> Personality of Mother Theresa

In fact, if you were to combine these qualities into one picture, the perfect caregiver must look like this:

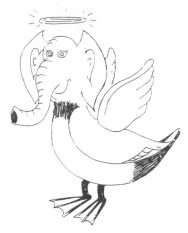

[My appreciation goes out to the family member of an Alzheimer's client who diligently worked to create this caricature.]

Even though comical, it is a very accurate description of those who are successful with the mentally impaired. The qualities represent:

1) *Part Elephant* - Caregivers must be "thick skinned" like an elephant. At times they can encounter both verbal and physical

outbursts from some mentally impaired clients. Caregivers must understand that the client's behavior is related to their impairment, and often their comments or reactions have little to do with the caregiver as an individual. To be "thick skinned" is to be able to experience these outbursts and not have it affect their relationship with the client.

2) *Part Duck* - There are days when caregivers will struggle with a client just to do basic care. Days where relating to this person is in itself the greatest challenge. Days where patience is stretched to its limit. However, by the next contact, or the next day, caregivers need to have virtually forgotten what happened and start fresh. They must have the ability to let things "roll off their backs" like water off a duck.

3) *Patience of a Saint* - To get certain clients to perform tasks or to understand what is required takes time, perseverance and patience. The qualities of any saint.

4) *Eyes of a Hawk* - Assessing a mentally impaired client requires caregivers to see things that are not easily visible to others. A caregiver's vision or insights must be as acute as a hawk. Constantly looking for the problem and adjusting their approach, based on what is found.

5) *Rationality of Mr. Spock* - At times caregivers need to be totally objective and rational. A realization that at times they just need to "do." If a client is incontinent and refuses to be changed, and no persuading, no cajoling seems to be effective, the reality is that the job has to be done now or it will never be done. An objective, rational approach with considerable tact like Mr. Spock from the movie Star Trek.

6) *Personality of Sister Theresa* - Staff require the compassion of Sister Theresa.

7) *Sense of Humor* - The ability to laugh is the primary skill of any effective caregiver and will often differentiate those who are successful from those who are not. Laughter is not at the expense of the client, but in response to the client's actions. For example, two caregivers can walk into the room of a dementia client and find him drawing pictures on the wall using his feces. One caregiver will fall to the floor with laughter saying "Well done Mr. Jones." The other caregiver becomes stern and upset saying to the first "How can you laugh over this?" The response by the first "I think he is doing a good job with the picture." The ability to laugh with the client can make our job bearable.

These descriptions profile those who possess the greatest amount of caring and compassion in dealing with this clientele, when mixed with the necessary knowledge, tools and skills their performance can excel.

Defining Priorities

I was asked to assess a unit housing a number of mentally impaired clients that demonstrated a great deal of disruptive wandering behavior. Based on my initial assessment of the unit, the lounge seemed to be the source of the problem. I established my plan of action - I would sit in the client's lounge to see how long I could last before I wanted to wander. The best vantage point was a two seat couch against one wall. A mentally impaired gentleman occupied one side of the couch. He was slumped over, staring at the floor (the care team later shared that this was his normal posture, he was usually expressionless and rarely communicated to anyone). I had no intention of maintaining a conversation with this man, only to assess the lounge. When I sat I said, "Hello" and then proceeded to watch the lounge.

After fifteen minutes of my sitting next to him, the man turned and stared at me. He stared for a good five minutes until he said "potatoes." I repeated to him "potatoes." For the next fifteen minutes this man talked to me about his potato farm of forty years ago - who worked on it, the problems he had, the money he made or lost, etc. During our conversation there was a dramatic shift in this man's posture and expression. He now sat erect, his face beamed and he grinned from ear-to-ear during the entire time we discussed his farm.

That was the end of my day, so I said good-bye to my new acquaintance and left the unit. I returned the next morning. When I walked past the nurse's station, I was accosted by the head nurse.

She said to me, "What did you do to that man last night?"

I said "I don't know, what did I do?"

She replied, "I don't know what you did either, but when you left last night, that client got up, got a hold of a waste paper basket and spent four hours wandering the unit looking for his potatoes. Don't do it again!"

I said, "Just a minute, was he a behavioral problem during that time? Was he disruptive, disturbing others?"

She responded, "No, he wasn't disturbing anyone. The problem was he wouldn't eat when he was supposed to eat, he wouldn't wash when he was supposed to wash and he wouldn't go to sleep when he normally does."

I asked, "After the four hours, did he eat, did he wash and did he go to bed?"

She answered. "Yes, he did."

And I returned, "*What was the problem?*"

If this nurse meant that I was not to allow this gentleman to experience anything positive because he disrupted her routine, then she has sadly missed the purpose of her role.

Quality of life is more than physical care. No matter what you do with the mentally impaired, whether positive or negative, it will have consequences. If you elicit from a mentally impaired individual something positive, then it may bring back memories that will elicit a change in behavior. Likewise, if you intensify the client's anxiety level, you may elicit agitation or wandering.

The goal of care is more complex than any medical model dealing with the symptoms of the disease. We have been charged with making the remainder of this person's life the most positive possible, given the limitations experienced. That may require our taking the person's symptoms and doing little more than making them tolerable to ourselves who do the care, and the other clients who must live with him. To emphasize only the physical aspects of this person's life brings us back to the days of custodial care, which is a frustrating environment for both caregivers and clients alike.

The Premise for Care

A number of years ago, when I was newly married and first a nurse, my wife and I accompanied thirty-five developmentally delayed children (i.e. Down's syndrome) to Florida for a two week vacation several years in a row. We were the nursing team along with fifteen counselors who organized and supervised the function.

Before our first venture, I had little contact with the developmentally challenged. My first two days were the most difficult. Being a newly graduated nurse, I believed I could change the world. In front of me now were a number of severely handicapped individuals whose behaviors were not unlike what we encounter with the mentally impaired elderly - spastic movements, repetitive speech, and so on.

On the second day, I finally dragged aside a counselor who had considerable experience with this clientele. I said to her, "Can't you see these children are having problems - considerable difficulty in their movements and speech? Why don't you do something to help them correct that?" I learned more on how to deal with our clientele from that person than from anyone else since.

She responded, "These children are developmentally challenged because of brain damage. There is nothing I can do to reverse the brain damage, therefore there is nothing I can do to stop the symptoms. My job is to look beyond the symptoms to see what is left of the person and then provide to the part that remains the greatest quality of life I can."

In caring for the mentally impaired elderly we unfortunately seem to place our emphasis more on the symptoms, than the person. The brain damage experienced by the mentally impaired cannot be reversed. Hence the premise for Supportive Therapy - identifying his strengths and maintaining them, his limitations and compensating for them, and intervene on the areas of vulnerability.

This means taking risks at times. No approach, environment or supportive measure works the same way all of the time for all of those who are mentally impaired. Our challenge is to determine which is the effective supportive measure during each moment of contact.

Caring for the mentally impaired is not an easy job. Nor is it a simple process to always be objective, constantly placing oneself behind the eyes of this client. There are times when those skills of being objective and empathetic are strained to their limit. It takes a "special" person to work with such a client experiencing "special" needs.

To be effective in providing care we must have clearly defined and enforced programs specifically geared to this individual and his limitations. If the challenge is met, we will ensure for this client that he will achieve the highest level of quality of life, living in an environment that is supportive - compensating for his limitations, enhancing his strengths and eliminating those things that target his vulnerabilities.

Chapter Eight

Understanding Behavior

This section is dedicated to understanding two common behaviors - wandering and sexual. The descriptions of each behavior includes:

- a list of the general causes for that behavior.
- a detailed description of each cause.
- the potential supportive measures to address each cause.

[Note: Aggression which is one of the most challenging behaviors is detailed in the book Preventing Alzheimer's Aggression: Supportive Therapy in Action.]

The causes presented are general categories only. Many categories can be divided into further sub-categories, i.e. the lifestyle category can include the client's past job, recreational past times, personality characteristics, individual likes and dislikes, etc. When analyzing the behavior it is beneficial to examine the causes in as much detail as possible to ensure accuracy in defining what may be causing the behavior and the required supportive measure.

There are references throughout this section to a number of behavior management tools presented in subsequent chapters - Care Analysis, Care Plan Summary, Diversional Measures, Retracting Measures, Redirecting Measures, Patterning, Programming Map, etc. Refer to the appropriate chapter if more detailed information on any of these tools is required.

The examples and case scenarios provided are long term care focused. Although these behaviors may be encountered to some degree in the community and acute care, they are common to long term care. To address the causative factors and supportive measures for all three specialties would make these chapters unwieldy. Those who work in acute care or the community will find it easy to extrapolate the information provided to make it specific to their specialty.

Wandering Behavior

The discussion on wandering behavior is divided into three parts:

> Part One: Potential Causes and Required Supportive Measures
> Part Two: The Wandering Path
> Part Three: Aggressive Elopement Behavior

Part One - Potential Causes and Required Supportive Measures

An overview of the potential causes for wandering include:

> Mimicking
> Looking for Something Familiar
> Investigative Wandering (Looking for blank)
> Fear/Anxiety/Stress
> Bored/Poor Attention Span
> Increased Energy
> Medication/Washroom Location
> Lifestyle
> External Cueing
> Physical Discomfort

Mimicking
Earlier we discussed how some mentally impaired clients can mimic almost any behavior if the stimulus is intense enough. The same is true with wandering behavior.

Defining the wandering path is a must. The wandering path is not only the physical layout of the unit, but the visible layout as well - the part of the hall or unit that attracts a mentally impaired client to it.

If the wandering path leads or attracts a client through a lounge, the results are self-evident. One wanderer will walk down the hall and into the lounge. Two mentally impaired clients will come out of the lounge and walk down the hall. On their return pass, they will both walk into the lounge. Three clients will then exit the lounge . . . Within a short time you could have up to six clients wandering all due to the activity of one.

Clients who are aware of the activity about them are the most susceptible. This individual can sit for extended periods of time if the environment is quiet and she is not distracted. If this client sees others walk past, then past again, she will be drawn to follow them. Once two clients are wandering the same path, others with a similar sensitivity are likely to follow.

Supportive Measure
1) Diversional Measure - Identifying the time of day when there is the greatest amount of wandering (utilizing Patterning), allows the caregiver to control the stimuli causing the behavior. Scheduling programming for chronic wanderers when they are the most active removes the stimuli for the mimicking client, or scheduling programming for the mimicking client during peak wandering activity removes the client from the stimuli (called Retracting Measures). In either case, the mimicking client is removed from the stimuli, decreasing the frequency of her behavior.

2) Eliminating Attractors - Shift change, tour groups, family visits, etc. will create a similar effect.

- If at shift change, the day and afternoon staff congregate at the nursing station (now referred to as the Information Station to create more of a team perspective) and the day staff leave the unit on mass, the mimicking client will probably follow them off the unit. It is important that stimuli affecting the mimicking client be controlled. The exodus of day staff from the unit should be invisible to the mentally impaired clients.

- A tour group of any type or size (i.e. professionals from another facility or organization, family of a perspective admission, contractors or repair people, etc.) will create the same results. The care team must be alerted when a tour group is scheduled to walk the unit in order to distract the mimicking client.

- The family admission package or orientation program should always educate family about the mimicking client (and other behaviors they may encounter). Family need direction on what to do if the mimicking client attempts to leave the unit with them; follow them and their family member while they walk the hall; or sit with them when they are in the lounge.

The more these attractors can be controlled, the less the mimicking client will wander.

3) Environmental Supports - Two or more lounges are needed on any unit that houses mentally impaired clients. Placing the mimicking client in a lounge out of view of the wandering path will eliminate the stimuli.

If only one large lounge is available (which is often the case in older facilities), then the mimicking client cannot help but wander. The floor plan (drawing #1) shows a common unit design in long term care, a long hallway with a large lounge at the end of the hall. The wandering path is obvious, the wanderer walks down the hall, into the lounge, is forced to turn around and walks out of the lounge.

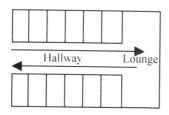

Drawing #1

Any client with mimicking tendency will be drawn to wander behind this individual.

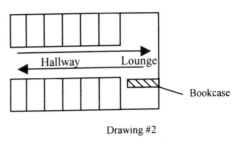

Drawing #2

The lounge can be divided into smaller private sitting areas to keep the mimicking client out of view of those who wander. Building a bookcase to divide the lounge (drawing #2) is an easy and inexpensive way to address this concern.

The bookcase is positioned to separate the lounge from the wandering path. The design of the bookcase is very specific (drawing #3). The bottom section of the book case contains the book shelves. However the upper section, from mid chest level to ceiling are 1 x 6 slats placed at an angle (drawing #4). This allows the client with mimicking tendencies to sit in the smaller room created by the book case divider. When caregivers are in the larger lounge area they are able to see through the slats to ensure that all is well in that room. The wandering client will walk into the main section of the lounge, turn to the book case, looking at the slats head on makes it appear as a solid wall, turn and walk back up the hall.

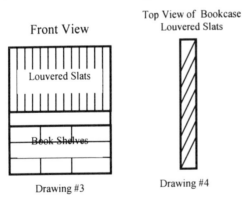

Front View

Louvered Slats

Book Shelves

Drawing #3

Top View of Bookcase
Louvered Slats

Drawing #4

A couple of additional points. Furniture or other objects (planters, pole lamp, etc.) should not be placed against the wall entering this additional room. Should the wanderer see objects near the entrance it may draw him into the sitting area to investigate, defeating the purpose of the room.

If there is a need to utilize the entire lounge for large group activities, then a piano hinge can be attached at the corner of the bookcase and to the wall, and a stabilizer pin attached to the end of the bookcase by the entrance to the sitting room. The pin is pushed down into a hole in the floor to secure it in place. When the entire lounge is to be used, the pin is pulled up and the bookcase pushed against the wall.

Although dividing a lounge may not be a need in every facility, there is another reason why this design was detailed. The louver slat design is ideal to camouflage any area or room. The angled slats allow the caregiver to see into that area, as well as optimum lighting and ventilation for the room. However, the mentally impaired do not have the cognitive ability to view through the angled slats. When they are standing in front of the divider, looking directly at the slats, it appears as a sold wall obscuring that area from view. An excellent fencing design for an enclosed courtyard.

Looking for Something Familiar

The need for the mentally impaired to find something familiar (spouse, house, clothing, etc.) to decrease anxiety was presented earlier. Wandering for this client is in response to the need to be constantly looking for specific objects (clothing, bedroom, etc.) or people (family members or friends). The Supportive Measures for this causative factor will be discussed with the next.

Investigative Wandering (Looking for blank)

Some have called this activity mere curiosity on the part of the mentally impaired. There is more to it than simple curiosity. Investigative wandering is common with clients who have poor recent memory retention but still maintain a degree of analytical ability or problem solving.

This is a client who does not know what she is looking for, no matter what she is given, it does not satisfy her. This individual walks around looking in every cupboard, drawer and/or behind every door. Once the client looks behind the door or inside the cupboard or drawer she can recognize what it is (retained analytical ability) which creates a degree of familiarity. As soon as she turns away from the door, cupboard or drawer she forgets what she saw (loss of recent memory) and continues to wander. When she returns to the same door, cupboard or drawer again she cannot remember what it is (loss of recent memory), she investigates it again and knows what it is (retained analytical ability). This client continually investigates her environment to create a sense of familiarity.

<u>Supportive Measures</u>
1) Wander - Each of these cases (looking for something familiar and investigative wandering) results in *random wandering*. Whenever a mentally impaired client decides that he must find something or his anxiety increases, he will wander. The best supportive measure is to let this client wander. To stop him is to increase his anxiety, and increase the possibility of an aggressive response. When he cannot wander he feels more confused, which elevates his anxiety even further. To wander gives him the feeling that he knows what is going on around him. However, allowing a mentally impaired client to wander freely requires a safe wandering environment (discussed later in this chapter).

2) Diversional Measure - Periodically intervening on this person's wandering may be necessary when the activity on the unit is excessive and the wandering is adding to the chaos; she is disturbing others; or the client herself is becoming exhausted and must be encouraged to sit in order to rest. Employing a diversional activity will distract her from her need to wander.

The length of time involved and/or the ability of the client to complete the task is an important indicator to her anxiety level and/or change in functioning ability. If the client is normally involved in a diversional task for fifteen minutes, anything less may be an indicator that something is different. Likewise, if the client is now having difficulty performing the task where performance was not an issue previously, something has changed.

Either there is a stressor or trigger elevating his anxiety,
requiring him to wander to decrease it
Or the disease has progressed decreasing his functioning ability,
making the task inappropriate.

It is important to focus on the individual's strengths as well as limitations. The inability to perform a task or function at a certain level can be an indictor that the disease has progressed or a new secondary factor has been introduced. In either case an assessment is needed to determine what is different and the new supportive measures required.

Fear/Stress/Anxiety

There are many examples where certain stimuli or circumstances cause an increase in fear, stress or anxiety among the mentally impaired (TV, aggressive outbursts by another client, group activity, etc.). Once the client's emotional state is elevated, the client wanders away from the potential source. Eliminate the stressor, and the wandering will be curtailed.

Supportive Measure

1) Remove the Stressor - Wandering caused by a specific stressor is often *patterned*. It virtually occurs the same time every day or as a result of the same stimuli or events. It is important to identify the pattern in order to determine the required supportive measure. Patterning is an assessment tool used to identify the time and event patterns of the behavior.

Patterning requires all caregivers to document a client's wandering by recording the time and "back tracking," describing what was occurring in the last location where he was sitting (an activity, aggressive outburst by another client, glare in the sitting room from bright sunlight, etc.). By reviewing what is documented, the care team may uncover a trend revealing what is causing this client's behavior and/or the time it is most common. For example, documentation describing four separate occasions reveals that wandering is generally around 1400 hours. "Back tracking" reveals that on each occasion the client was sitting in the lounge and a recreational activity was conducted in that lounge at 1330 hours. This client was not directly involved in that activity. The care team surmised that the client was unable to handle the stimuli created by that event. In order to intervene on this client's behalf, it was necessary to relocate the client before the activity begins or to re-locate the activity to another room.

2) Addressing the Time Factor - Always finding the stressor or cause may not be easy. The descriptions of what was happening around or to the client may reveal no pattern. However, knowing the time pattern is valuable. If the client wanders everyday around 1400 hours, then a diversional activity of some type prior to that time would remove her from the stressor experienced even though it has not been uncovered, decreasing the need to wander.

Bored, Poor Attention Span, Restlessness

These are all related. A client with poor recent memory may also have a poor attention span and as a result become very restless. This individual easily loses track of what is happening, finding most activities or events confusing. This results in the client becoming bored, increasing his restlessness, encouraging him to wander.

If the wandering path in which he walks is too complicated, posing many blind bluffs and turns, he can easily become confused. Not knowing where he is going, he then sits in the first empty chair he can find. Again, his poor attention span results in his sitting in that chair for a few moments. He becomes bored and restless, stands and begins to wander again. Finding the first empty chair he comes to (which may be the one he just left), he sits . . . He continues that activity throughout the day. This type of wandering can be called *Stop/Go Wandering*.

Supportive Measures

1) Bursts of Activity - This client is responding to his restlessness by moving from one chair to another. His activity does not exhaust his increasing energy level, and as a result does nothing to alleviate his

problem. The only practical supportive measure is to provide bursts of activity every hour to an hour and a half, in order to decrease his restlessness and eliminate the need for the stop/go wandering.

A common response to such a suggestion is that it cannot be done. Time and staffing restraints make it impossible to implement such an intervention. Their assessment of the actual situation is totally inaccurate. These supportive measures are common, unfortunately in some settings it often depends who is on duty at the time, whether it is done or not.

Those with a poor attention span are usually early risers. Once they are awake, the night shift knows they will not go back to sleep. These clients are often dressed and placed in the lounge, rather than being forced to stay in bed and sleep. This means that the housekeeper, who usually cleans the lounge the first thing in the morning when few clients are there, probably meets these clients nearly every morning. If the housekeeper on duty understands the mentally impaired, she is often doing what is required.   Knowing that these clients are restless, she turns on the radio to get them singing and dancing at the same time she is cleaning. That housekeeper has just provided the needed burst of activity to decrease the restlessness of those clients and eliminate their need to wander.

The same is true with nursing staff. If the right staff member is on duty, she is usually providing bursts of activity to the clients who need it as well. She will often encourage specific clients to follow her at certain times of the day, asking them to carry laundry or push a cart under supervision. This is sound problem solving.

Clients cannot afford hit/miss programming - where what is done is dictated by who is on duty. It is important that the care team identify the clients who fit this criteria - low attention span, easily bored, restless. Once identified, the efforts of all team members must be coordinated so that these clients receive bursts of activity scheduled every hour. This requires:

- the housekeeper responsible to clean the lounge to get these clients moving for about five minutes.

- the clients care routine (washing, breakfast, bathing, grooming and other activities) must be scheduled throughout the morning rather than concentrated during one time period.
- recreation staff need to conduct five minute exercise sessions with these clients or power walk them when she is available.
- volunteer or family visits coordinated to fill in the times not covered.

A programming schedule for this client's day would appear as follows (recorded on the Daily Log section of the Care Plan Summary):

0700 - Singing with housekeeper in the lounge
0800 - Breakfast
0900 - Grooming
1000 - Power walk with Recreation
1100 - Gather laundry with nursing staff
1200 - Lunch
1300 - Assist laundry staff
1400 - Family visit

This simple programming strategy decreases the client's restlessness, and possibly eliminates much of the stop/go wandering behavior.

Increased Energy

This is one of the most challenging individuals. Metabolism seems to be in high gear for this client resulting in the following behavioral characteristics:

- constant and fast paced wandering.
- sleeping only short periods.
- unable to sit for a meal.
- rapid weight loss.
- takes short rest periods, staying in a chair for only a few moments at a time.

This client demonstrates two levels of wandering - controlled and uncontrolled. Controlled wandering is where the person is still able to maneuver the environment, walking around objects or people. An uncontrolled state is when this client's energy is at its peak and he is unable to maneuver around objects or people. Anything or anyone in his way will be pushed along or pushed aside. Frail clients in this individual's path during periods of uncontrolled wandering are at risk of being injured.

Supportive Measures
1) Patterning - It is important to define the times when this client's energy is at its greatest (uncontrolled wandering period). These times are usually of a short duration. The client does not have sufficient energy to keep up that pace for extended periods. Once the peak energy level is exhausted, the client will return to his normal pace (controlled wandering). During these peak times the person must be power walked. The individual attempting to walk with him will have trouble keeping up, however the purpose of the power walk is to maneuver him around objects and people until he is able to maneuver on his own.

2) Caloric Intake - Energy drinks and frequent meals of finger foods (foods he can eat on the run) are essential to control the weight loss caused by the constant movement (a physician and dietician should be consulted for the required drinks and foods). It is important to note that regardless of the caloric intake, weight loss is inevitable. Once the weight loss reaches a critical point, the client will no longer be able to walk. The wandering will have stopped to be replaced by a new behavior - continually rocking in the chair to expel the energy build-up.

The Disease Process (Repetitive Behavior)

Chronic wandering by some mentally impaired clients may be caused by the persistent stimuli effect described earlier. In these cases, biological changes within the brain causes this client to walk continuously. This is different than wandering due to increased energy. In the above situation the person had to wander to expel the energy build-up. In this case the person cannot stop walking but does not have the energy to maintain the constant movement. As the day progresses, this client becomes exhausted, increasing her risk for frequent falls.

Supportive Measures
1) Rest Periods - It is imperative to determine the length of time this client can wander before she is tired and having difficulty with her balance. When she is tired, she will need to be placed in a chair for a period to allow her to rest. An effective chair is either a recliner or a chair with the back legs shortened by three inches. In either of these chairs, she will find it difficult to get up on her own (due to the apraxia discussed earlier). She may try to get up when first placed in the chair, but she will often succumb to her exhaustion and nap in the chair. When she awakes and is restless again, she needs to be allowed to wander until her next rest period. Patterning determines the times when she is tired and when these rest periods should be scheduled.

Medications & Location of The Washroom
The two drugs that frequently cause wandering behavior with the mentally impaired elderly are diuretics and laxatives. The sensitivity of the mentally impaired elderly to medication is well defined. A mentally impaired older client on a laxative or diuretic will always have the feeling that "he has to go." If he is aware of the need and afraid of being incontinent, he will continually wander in order to find the washroom.

Supportive Measures
1) Visible Washroom - Having a washroom visible from the wandering path will not only decrease the amount and frequency of wandering, but will also decrease the frequency of incontinence. The majority of mentally impaired clients recognize a toilet (ingrained long term memory). Wandering a hallway and seeing a toilet will often result in a dementia client walking in and using it.

Some are concerned about the lack of privacy for a dementia client using a toilet that is visible to the hallway. If the toilet is not visible then the client will be incontinent or required to wear an incontinent brief. It is not uncommon for mentally impaired clients wearing an incontinent brief to remove them to urinate in a chair, on a tree in the lounge (male client), in a waste paper basket, in a corner of the room, on a radiator (male client). If an incontinent brief is not used, then the client is forced to walk the unit with a wet dress or pants. Whether an incontinent brief is used or not, the client will still have to be changed which often creates an aggressive response.

No one questions the emphasis to make every setting disabled accessible. It is expected then any location housing those with physical disabilities would be designed to accommodate those individuals and ensure their independence - a larger washroom, hand rails, ramps. The same philosophy must hold true with locations housing the mentally impaired elderly. The unit (or home) must be adapted to the strengths and limitations of the client. Individuals who visit those locations must be educated on what to expect and how to respond to the special needs of this client. Should a dementia client be seen using the washroom visible to the hallway, whoever encounters this situation (staff of all departments, family members and other regular visitors) should be instructed to draw the privacy curtain. Should the privacy curtain still be drawn across the door of the washroom when no one is in there, then whoever discovers it should simply pull it back so the next dementia client walking by has a clear view of the toilet.

2) Environmental Cues - Unfortunately, the layout of a client's bedroom can cause wandering. A common room in a health care facility has three doors - hallway, closet and bathroom. If the bathroom and closet doors are closed, the client will maintain his ritualistic patterned behavior and go into the hallway (the most common door he uses) to look for the bathroom. Removing the bathroom door so the toilet is always visible and placing locator signs (on the door frame of the bathroom, and on the closet door) indicating by picture and word what is in that room or behind the closet will decrease the need to search.

3) Night Light - Family must be asked how often their family member goes to the bathroom during the night. It is common for the elderly to go to the washroom one or more times during the night. Placing a night light in the washroom that shines on the toilet prevents the need to walk into the hallway looking for the washroom. A high/low bed that lowers to nine inches (twenty-three centimeters) from the floor, allows the bed to be at a height where the client can rise safely and without assistance.

4) Incontinence Program - Time patterning incontinence or night wandering is valuable to indicate when the bladder is full and must empty. An Incontinence Program attempts to determine when a client must be assisted to the toilet to avoid incontinence. If the client is normally incontinent and awake at 0200 hours, then he should be checked the next night at 0145 hours. If he is incontinent at that time, then he should be checked the next night at 0130 hours. If he is still dry, then he needs to be toileted (commode chair or walked to the toilet) and then returned back to bed. Toileting him every night at 0130 hours creates a care routine that responds to his physical needs. Of course monitoring the amount of fluids taken before bedtime and toileting him just prior to bedtime will decrease the need to wake him at 0130 hours.

Some believe that the client should be left to sleep and simply allowed to be incontinent in his incontinent briefs. That statement 'allowed to be incontinent' is a contradiction to client centered care and quality care practices. Incontinent briefs should only be used as a safeguard against the person being incontinent or for individuals who have lost physical control of bladder function. The practice of using incontinent briefs on individuals with bladder control rather than an Incontinence Program should always be questioned. Incontinence with or without incontinent briefs should be avoided where possible. Having to change a dementia client will often result in aggressive behavior, crying out, restlessness and/or wandering behavior. The care routine compensates for the client's limitations in every other aspect of care - assists those who are unable to feed, dress or bath themselves. The care routine must also assist those who are unable to toilet themselves.

5) Sensory Lighting - Sensory lighting in washrooms and the hallway has become a valuable supportive device for those clients who are up during the night. However, having the sensor that turns on the bathroom light located in the washroom is of little value. The client has to walk into the washroom for the light to turn on. Locating the sensor for the washroom light outside of the bathroom, turns the washroom light on when the client walks by the bathroom door, drawing the client into the washroom.

6) High Tech - Many computerized supportive devices that benefit dementia clients are now available:

- Incontinent pads with a computerized sensor signals a caregiver's beeper when a client is incontinent. This prevents the need to physically check the client during rounds or to wait for the client to become restless, wander or call out. The main computer also stores the times when the client has been incontinent and then analyzes the information to define the time the caregiver should toilet the client to prevent him from being incontinent.
- Room sensors signal a caregiver's beeper to indicate that a client is up who should not be up.
- Room sensor delays allow the client to be up without setting off the sensor, should the person not return to bed in the prescribed time, a caregiver's beeper is activated to check on the client.

This is only the beginning. Computerized devices will assist in developing accurate client centered care practices and routines. It will be interesting to see the response by some caregivers as these tools are introduced.

Lifestyle

An important question to ask the family of a mentally impaired client is:

How has your father (mother) dealt with stress all of his (her) life?

Their answer will provide considerable insight into their father's behavior now. If family state that in the past their father dealt with his stress by walking it off, then his constant wandering probably does the same now. It is important then to let him wander and investigate what may be causing the distress.

Supportive Measure

1) Personal History - Past lifestyle is a common contributor to present behavior. One male client demonstrated chronic and sometimes agitated wandering. All previous efforts to distract him from his incessant, non-directed wandering failed. The only history on this client was that he had been a laborer for the past thirty-eight years. The care team did not experience success until after his family told them an interesting point about their father's past employment. The family revealed that their father had been a sweeper for the past twenty years. Wandering was his life.

Immediately upon receiving that information, the care team gave this client a broom and encouraged him to sweep the hallway. From that point on his wandering became directed and his agitation was completely eliminated. Each day he would find some debris on the floor and chase it around the unit with his broom. More importantly, he was now more cooperative to stop for his lunch. Furthermore, he could be persuaded to put his broom away by late afternoon and sit in the lounge for a extended period of time. If he saw some dirt in the hallway, he would get his broom, chase the dirt around the unit for awhile, and then return his broom back to its closet. The care team successfully changed a disruptive behavior into something that was now tolerable.

A further footnote about this gentleman. He often displayed an interesting behavior while he was sweeping. He would now stop what he was doing to have a brief conversation with anyone who approached him. Something that was contrary to his behavior before he was given the broom. Standing in the hallway, he would talk to the person while he leaned on his broom with his right elbow, and stroked his chin with his left hand (something he probably did throughout his twenty years as a sweeper).

Programming that relates to the client's personal history is frequently a successful supportive measure to address many behaviors (refer to the subsequent chapter on Programming).

2) Triggers or Stressors - If the client has always used walking to deal with stress, then his wandering now is an indicator of a possible stressor. Utilizing patterning, the care team can now use his wandering to uncover the stressor (TV, large group activity, aggressive outbursts by another client, etc.) and determine the needed Retracting Measure to remove him from the stressor or the stressor from him.

3) Activity Centers - These are environmental attractors that will hold the dementia client's attention. Discussed in the chapter on Programming, activity centers are located in view of the wandering path and 'hook' a client's past memory - carpenter center, sewing center, gardening center and so on. Investigating the center and manipulating the related objects located at the center decreases the frequency and duration of a client's wandering.

External Cueing/Attractors
Spring can create a significant amount of wandering activity on any long term care unit. Being indoors all winter, and then experiencing a beautiful April day creates a desire to be out in the sun.

On one unit, housekeeping staff found that the clutter and activity in the hallway made it difficult to wash the hallway floor with the power mobile washer during the day. They decided (without consultation with the care team) to use the power mobile washer later in the evening when most of the clients were in the room. As the power washer tracked up and down the hall, more and more ambulatory mentally impaired clients would peek out their bedroom door to investigate what it was. Once in the hallway they began wandering the unit.

Wandering due to external cueing is different than mimicking wandering. Where the mimicking wanderer follows the stimuli, wandering due to external cueing is drawn to investigate the stimuli, unable to return to the original location or activity, the client wanders as a result. A PA system, a loud TV down the hall, people talking in a room, equipment noises, etc. will create this effect.

Supportive Measures

1) Timing of Events - Everything and anything can effect a dementia client and impact on care delivery. No department or individual can work unilaterally without negatively impacting on the client and care delivery. Scheduling the use of floor polishers and washers, conducting maintenance repairs, large group activities, tour groups, etc. must be planned based on the sensitivities of the client who live in that setting. If the scheduling of certain activities cannot accommodate the unit, then the care team must always be given warning in advance of what will occur so they can plan what must be done to distract the sensitive client (proactive care) rather than intervene when the client's behavior is demonstrated (reactive care).

2) Controlling Stimuli - The care team must have the freedom and authority to delay or even cancel specific activities if the dementia clients on a unit are over-stimulated. Keeping the status quo when a unit is "wired" or specific clients are unmanageable is a total disrespect for the clients who live there and the caregivers who work there. There is no status quo when caring for the dementia client. Care and activities must be flexible to needs of the client.

Physical Discomfort

Many older clients suffer from arthritis or joint pain. Any physical discomfort - pain, constipation, hunger, thirst, feeling cold or too hot, etc. may cause a mentally impaired client to wander in reaction to those needs.

Supportive Measures

1) Pain Management - Each of the following has the potential of decreasing wandering behavior (note: it is important that a physician be consulted before any medication is given):

- Dispensing a mild analgesic such as enteric coated aspirin or an anti-inflammatory medication decreases joint pain.
- A common symptom for anyone under stress is an upset stomach due to excessive gastric excretion. We have identified frequently the stress associated with dementia. Wandering that occurs two hours after a meal can indicate gastric distress. Dispensing an antacid will relieve gastric pain and decrease wandering behavior.
- Any client who has a history of hemorrhoids and is not receiving ointment for the relief of hemorrhoid discomfort will tend to wander.

2) Environmental Supports - Available snacks, appropriate temperature control, control of noise level, etc. will all have the potential to decrease wandering behavior.

Part Two - The Wandering Path

Some will say, "Why not just let all of the clients who want to wander, wander?" In some situations that is the most appropriate supportive measure. The decision to intervene on wandering behavior depends on what is causing it. Like aggression and almost all other behaviors of the mentally impaired, wandering may be a symptom of an underlying problem. The intervention needed depends on the problem causing it (see chapter on Care Analysis).

For some clients, there is no intervention available that will stop or decrease their wandering, and for others there is. Excessive wandering by a number of clients on any unit can create significant problems:

1) Mimic wandering - clients who are capable of concentrating on a specific task can be distracted by the constant stimuli of seeing others wander, and as a result, are unable to complete the task.

2) Indiscriminate wandering - it is difficult to monitor a large number of clients who wander at one time. The more who wander, the more who will walk into other client's rooms; rummage through other client's things; bump into others; block the entrances, doors and walking paths, etc. only increasing the incidents of aggressive outbursts on the unit.

3) Lineal wandering - walking up and down a hall with no change in direction (pacing) can cause an increase in anxiety and agitation.

4) Increased risk of elopement behavior - the more clients who are wandering, the more who are attempting to leave the building.

5) Forced wandering - the more clients wandering, the greater risk that some clients will be virtually dragged out of their chairs by wandering clients wanting them to follow. This increases the incidents of aggressive outbursts and places a not too stable client at risk of falling.

The list goes on. Wandering must be safe and minimized so that it does not disrupt other clients, and will not result in the person being injured or injuring others. To accomplish this, there are a number of options that can be employed when dealing with wandering behavior.

1) The Physical Wandering Path

The most appropriate wandering path provides directional change. Any unit that is shaped in a "U" or in a circle would accomplish that effect. Directional change eliminates a sense of covering the same territory over and over again. Lineal wandering, or wandering up and down a straight corridor can increase agitation. It is more akin to pacing, and can create a "caged in" feeling.

If the unit can only provide a lineal wandering path, then the care team need to define the client's endurance level:

Endurance level - how long before the wanderer becomes agitated.

Some mentally impaired clients can wander up and down the same corridor every day, all day long and not experience any difficulty. Others can tolerate pacing the hall for only a short time before they feel trapped. Once that feeling is experienced, anxiety can increase causing an agitated response.

A client's endurance level is defined by Patterning. If the client demonstrates increased agitation after an hour of pacing, then the client's recreational activities and care routine must be scheduled to cover every hour of this person's day (defined by the Programming Map and outlined in the Care Plan Summary). This will allow a break in that client's wandering pattern. As discussed earlier, implementing these supportive measures require a coordinated effort by the entire care team.

2) Creating a Safe Wandering Environment

Elopement behavior is a mentally impaired client's attempt to leave a unit or the building.

There are two types of elopement behavior. One is the *aggressive eloper*, this is the client who makes a "bee line" for the nearest exit and once outside is difficult to return to the building. The other is the *incidental eloper*, the client who is found wandering aimlessly out in the yard and is easy to return to the unit.

The incidental eloper is often drawn out of the building by some external stimuli. For example, a mentally impaired client may be drawn to an exit door in the wandering path. If through the window in that door she sees a nice sunny day; a shopping mall down the street; a garden that needs to be tended; people walking along the sidewalk; etc. she may be attracted to that stimuli and walk out the door. She is not intending to leave but just drawn outside. Once outside, the door locks when it closes behind her. She then wanders aimlessly until someone returns her back to the unit.

The same dynamics will occur if a wandering client sees a stairwell as he walks past a door. Once he sees the stairs, he will go down for a simple reason - to see where they go (*the mentally impaired are always looking for something familiar and investigating the environment to decrease their anxiety*). Rarely will a mentally impaired client walk up the stairs. You will more often find them walking down. The common reason they will walk down, rather than up is often due to progressive apraxia. To travel up the stairs, requires considerable muscle coordination and strength. To travel down the stairs, one just follows gravity.

One of the best ways to ensure safe wandering is to secure exterior and stairwell doors. Buzzers are of little value. They will be activated regardless of who opens the door. Any door where there is significant traffic will be activated constantly. A magnetic security device solves many problems. Although most long term care facilities now secure exit doors in this manner, many acute care units do not. However, the wandering dementia client is also found on these units. Securing unit doors where this client is located is the only way to address the safety and liability risk that is present.

The magnetic security device works on the same principle as the magnetic fire door closures. Fire doors in hallways of most facilities are propped open against electronic magnets on the walls. The magnet, when it is activated, holds the fire doors open, allowing easy access and ventilation. The source of power to those magnets is connected to the fire alarm system. When the fire alarm sounds or the power goes off, the magnets automatically shut off, releasing the fire doors and they close tight.

The magnetic security device works under the same principle, but in reverse. An electronic magnet attached to the door frame of an exit door holds the door closed. When someone wants to leave or enter the unit, that person needs to push in and hold a button on the wall. Once the button is pressed, it deactivates the magnet and releases the door, allowing the person to open the door. Once the button is released, the magnet is reactivated automatically, securing the door as soon as it closes.

The power to this magnet is also connected to the fire alarm system. When the fire alarm sounds or the power goes off, the magnet is deactivated and the door can be opened freely. With this device, the door is not locked, but only secured, making it nearly impossible for the mentally impaired to open it and leave the unit.

Another security device that is even more complex is the numbered magnetic security system. It works on the same principle as what was just described. The difference is that instead of having one button, there is a box with six buttons, each numbered from one to six. A person coming onto the unit needs to only turn the handle on the door, the magnet is automatically deactivated. To leave the unit, a specific number sequence must be pushed to release the magnet so the door can be opened. Again, if the fire alarm sounds or the power goes off, the magnet automatically shuts off and the door can be opened freely.

To allow visitors, family members, cognitively well clients and other staff to freely come and go from the unit, it is important to place a sign near the door with instructions on how to deactivate the magnetic device. A mentally impaired client will be unable to read the instructions, understand what they mean, push the button and have the manual dexterity to open the door at the same time. If that client is capable of following those instructions and open the door, then his degree of impairment must be questioned.

One last point on using this device. If the button that deactivates the lock is a black button, surrounded by a silver wall cover, located on a brown wall, then there will be another problem. Some of your mentally impaired clients will be attracted to that wall plate, pushing it over and over again (*if the stimulus is too intense, some mentally impaired cannot help but respond*). A simple solution is to wallpaper the wall, as well as the silver cover, with a pattern of black-eyed Suzies. To the mentally impaired the button is lost in a sea of black buttons (*if the stimulus is not intense enough it will be missed or misinterpreted*) and they will no longer be attracted to it.

There are two additional supportive measures that will often prevent dementia clients from walking off the unit or into any side rooms (office, supply room, etc.). One way is to place a "smoke" film over glass windows or place sheers over the door windows at the end of the hall or to any side rooms. The darkened glass will appear solid black to the mentally impaired (*if the stimulus is not intense enough, it will be missed or misinterpreted*), keeping the exterior or stairwells from view, decreasing the tendency to be drawn through the door. The second option is to paint the door and door frame the same color as the wall. This camouflages the door, making it invisible to the mentally impaired.

One last point on creating a safe wandering path. The wanderer must have available to him visible resting areas scattered throughout. These could be small alcoves where a couple of comfortable chairs and a small end table are located. In this way the wanderer is provided an opportunity to rest during his journey.

3) Securing an Elevator

It is always interesting to see the color elevators are painted on units that house the mentally impaired. Often the walls are beige and the elevator is bright blue. That is the technique used to make client rooms stand out - paint the door frames a bright color in contrast to the wall. To hide the elevator, it need only be painted the same color as the wall. That will make it virtually invisible, preventing the mentally impaired from being attracted to it.

The elevator can still be a problem. On the wall next to the elevator is a steel plate with two buttons. The mentally impaired will be attracted to the plate and buttons, pushing one often by accident. The elevator is summoned; the door opens; the client is attracted inside the elevator; the door closes; the elevator proceeds to the next floor; the door opens again; and the client walks out and wanders about on another floor.

A simple solution is to place a metal plate over the two buttons. Two holes are pre-drilled in the plate, one over each of the buttons.

The holes must be smaller than an adult's little finger. Anchored to the wall next to the plate is a small chain. Attached to the end of the chain is a stick which is the exact diameter of the holes in the plate. To summon the elevator, one only needs to slip the stick through one of the holes and depress the button. The mentally impaired will be unable to use such a complex device. They can no longer summon the elevator on their own. (Note: Modern elevators can be set so that both the up and down button must be pushed at the same time to summon the elevator. A task the mentally impaired cannot complete.)

Two supportive measures have been presented, one that prevents the mentally impaired from being drawn to the elevator by its color, and the other from accidentally summoning the elevator by pushing the buttons. A third potential problem still remains. This occurs when the elevator doors open on their own as a mentally impaired client passes. If someone summoned the elevator and walked away, or if there are two elevators and both arrive on the unit when the button is pushed, the client sees the doors open and will inadvertently walk in. To prevent this from occurring, a black mat can be placed on the floor in front of the elevator.

The rationale for using the black mat is based on the perceptual difficulties experienced by the mentally impaired. Many mentally impaired clients have difficulty interpreting color changes experienced on the floor. One facility demonstrated this well. The hall consisted of white floor tiles with a black border lining the wall. The black border ran across the entrance to the dining room. Caregivers had considerable difficulty getting certain mentally impaired clients to cross the threshold into the dining room. When these clients reached the door and saw the black strip, they would stop, requiring staff to coax them to continue. When the client proceeded through the door, clients would inadvertently raise their foot to step over the black line. Those black lines represented a hole or a step (*if the stimulus is not intense enough, it will be missed or misinterpreted*) and the client was unsure of how to cross over.

The black mat creates the same effect. Some have tried these mats in front of exit doors, but found that they are usually not successful. If placed in front of an exit door, it may stall the mentally impaired from proceeding, but it will not stop them. They will reach the mat, place one foot on it to test it, then another foot and another until they reach the door. When placed in front of an elevator the black mat is most effective. It is easy to demonstrate.

The client is walking past the elevator just as the doors are opening. The person turns to walk in, sees the mat and stops. Not sure of what it is, he will take one step on the mat to test it, then another and another. By the time he reaches the elevator door, it will have closed and he will walk away.

Part Three - Aggressive Elopement Behavior

There are few mentally impaired clients who are true aggressive elopers. The aggressive eloper is one who heads for any exit door he can find, and makes a "bee line" down the street. Once the client has left the building, he is not easy to return and can become agitated at any attempt. Often the experience by caregivers with this client makes them uncomfortable to approaching him alone, resulting in two caregivers running after him.

When not trained to deal with such an occurrence, caregivers can exasperate the situation - approaching the client from behind, grab him by the arm in an attempt to turn him around to lead him back to the building. His response to such an approach is to become aggressive for two reasons.

1) Even though he is mentally impaired, he still knows that he is being turned around.
2) Having two people he does not know approach him in that manner will only result in his defending himself.

When caregivers discover that a client has walked away from the building, their strategy must be well planned. If two caregivers may be needed, one should approach the client from one side of the street and the other from the opposite side. When the one on the same side of the street reaches the client, she must circle around to the client's dominant side and approach at an angle to be in his field of vision and not block his path. That caregiver needs to smile at the client and carry on a conversation of an appropriate topic he can relate to in order to relax him and enhance rapport or trust in her. The other caregiver should remain on the other side of the street, ready to approach when called upon. Abrupt change in direction must be avoided. The client should be guided around the block or a parking lot and then back to the facility. The mentally impaired will not be aware of the direction change and will willingly lead back to the facility. This approach strongly increases the likelihood of returning to the facility with the least amount of aggression.

It is important that the care team use the eloper's exiting as an excuse to assess the environment. If it was that easy for a client to leave the building, then steps must be taken to adapt the environment to prevent it from occurring again (as discussed earlier).

Chapter Nine

Sexual Behavior

There is no more delicate topic than sex,
especially sexual activity of the dementia client.

The more restrictive an individual's ideation regarding specific sexual language or acts, the more difficult it is to maintain objectivity when witnessing those acts or hearing that language. Sexual behavior has the potential to challenge caregivers in a number of ways:

- Personal Values
- Society's Sensitivities
- Personal/Professional Education
- Caregiver Personal History

Understanding what creates restrictive beliefs is important before sexual behavior of the dementia client can be discussed.

Values
Certain sexual acts or language has the potential to challenge some religious, cultural, familial and/or personal values. The following are a few examples of these values and how they may influence a caregiver's response to the sexual behavior of a dementia client.

1) Religious Values - Some religions consider certain sexual acts, words or language sinful. Individuals who maintain strong religious beliefs may have difficulty maintaining their objectivity when those acts, words or language are encountered. It is difficult for some to deem these as sinful in

every situation, but abandon those beliefs in isolated instances despite the fact that it involves a dementia client.

2) Culture - In any multi-cultural society there is the potential for cultural conflicts. It is common in certain middle east cultures for two men to greet by kissing each other on both cheeks. However in a western culture such an act between two men would have a very different connotation or meaning. When a dementia client from a middle east culture approaches a male caregiver, visitor or other male client in this way it could be misunderstood.

3) Familial - Some caregivers have difficulty with physical affection even with their own family (i.e. hugging, kissing, etc.). When a caregiver finds physical affection difficult, it is hard to accept such contact from a dementia client.

4) Personal - Each person has a personal territory, the physical distance someone can approach before one feels intimidated or uncomfortable. This distance varies depending on the level of intimacy or relationship the other person is held. A dementia client does not recognize the territory of others and will approach someone at what can be considered an intimidating or intimate manner.

The more rigid a caregiver's beliefs, the more difficult it is to accept the sexual behavior of others regardless of the source or reason behind that behavior. Those caregivers who possess more liberal sexual values can be more accepting of the dementia client and at times confused by the actions or response by fellow caregivers who become distressed or judgmental when they witness the same sexual behavior.

Society's Sensitivity
Society's sensitivity towards sexual abuse and harassment is much different today then it was only a few years ago. It is refreshing that

the legal system finally recognizes the severity of such an assault regardless of when it occurred. However, those with restrictive sexual ideation may view the high profile of sexual harassment and abuse as justification for their own beliefs, classifying the sexual behavior of the dementia client as harassment or abuse and believing that some form of punitive action should be taken.

Personal/Professional Education

Each caregiver varies in their personal and professional education and experience with sexual behavior. Some caregivers can be described as 'street smart', individuals who have experienced a variety of challenging situations. The language and actions of the dementia client are tame in comparison to what they have encountered in their life. Other caregivers encounter certain sexual acts, language and words for the first time when caring for those with dementia. They can become flustered by what they experience, having difficulty maintaining their objectivity.

Combine this with the fact that professionals vary in their ability to understand a client's sexual behavior. Until recently, few health care professionals were formally trained on sexual behavior. The care team looks to those who are professionally trained (i.e. registered staff) for direction. When the registered staff are no better equipped to understand or address the behavior, they may react or make decisions based on their personal beliefs, misdirecting the care team in their approach or response to the client.

Caregiver Personal History

Caregivers who have been sexually used or abused are sensitive to the actions of others. It would be difficult for a caregiver to maintain objectivity if the dementia client uses similar words, voice tone or mannerisms as the person who abused or used them.

Each of these issues has the potential to influence a caregiver's reaction to the sexual behavior of a dementia client. The more restrictive the ideation, the more limiting the caregiver's objectivity. The belief that mentally impaired clients are incapable of comprehending their actions and behavior when it comes to all tasks of daily living <u>except</u> sexual behavior must continually be challenged. Any discussion or training regarding sexual behavior must also include the personal challenges that each caregiver may face.

Sexually Expressive Behavior

Sexual expressive behavior will be discussed in two parts:

Part One - Dynamics of Sexual Expressive Behavior
Part Two - Causes and Supportive Measures

Part One - Dynamics of Sexual Expressive Behavior

The mentally impaired express their sexual needs no differently than they express any other. If a dementia client experiences significant anxiety, she will probably become aggressive or withdraw. If a client needs to urinate, he will urinate. Likewise if a sexual need arises, a client will respond to that need.

Sexual behavior by the dementia client should not be considered or categorized as inappropriate. To classify sexual behavior of the dementia client as inappropriate is to imply that the person knows what he is doing and is doing it intentionally. Those with dementia do not have the cognitive ability to comprehend their actions. Using the word inappropriate to describe any behavior by a dementia client is inaccurate and validates the restrictive sexual ideation of some caregivers. The term sexually expressive behavior is more applicable. It is an expressive behavior used to communicate a need. Define the need or causative factor, implement the appropriate supportive measure and it will be possible to manage the behavior.

a) Sexual Intercourse
Level two mentally impaired clients are often unable to penetrate for sexual intercourse or masturbate to ejaculation. A common

comment expressed by a spouse of a mentally impaired client is, "My husband will talk about sex, we begin fondling each other, but we never complete it." It is not the lack of physical ability that restricts performance, but mental dysfunctioning.

Sexual intercourse requires considerable concentration and memory retention. Level two mentally impaired clients are incapable of maintaining that level of cognitive functioning. When the act is initiated, it is easily forgotten.

It is common for a spouse to be confused by the actions of their mate. The frequent invitation to resume their sexual activity can become frustrating when it is not completed, placing further stress on the relationship. Addressing the sexual behavior of the dementia client in a family information package, a family support group and/or family education session will greatly assist family members to understand the behavior and maintain their objectivity

b) Masturbation

The dynamics regarding sexual intercourse also apply to masturbation. A male dementia client may have an erection, fondle himself, but rarely complete to ejaculation. His short term memory loss and minimal attention span will prevent him from completing the act.

Masturbation should not be the issue. A client fondling him or herself out of sight of others is of no concern. However, the fact that the mentally impaired are oblivious to those around them often results in dementia clients exposing themselves and masturbating in some very public places.

Our primary goal is to maintain a client's dignity. In this instance the required supportive measure is to direct the client to a more private location. However, intervening after the individual has exposed himself is of little value. The focus must be proactive. The need to masturbate often presents some form of pre-emptive cueing, a pre-warning sign that the behavior will soon commence. Once the pre-emptive cue is witnessed (pulling on his zipper, raising her skirt, fondling oneself, etc.), the client needs to be relocated to his/her room.

This is not the responsibility of nursing staff only. The pre-emptive cueing must be communicated to all in regular contact with any unit housing dementia clients (see Care Plan Summary), including managers, staff of all departments, volunteers and regular family visitors. Volunteers and regular family visitors are not told that the client will masturbate when the pre-emptive cue is witnessed (confidentiality must be maintained), only that these actions need to be brought to the attention of the care team.

Some are surprised that regular family visitors would be included in this discussion. Regular family visitors are often in the client's lounge for extended periods of time, without this information family are left to witness a client masturbating resulting in their:

- visits becoming uncomfortable and potentially less frequent.
- becoming further stressed knowing that their family member is subjected to this behavior.
- mistakenly believing that the care team does not take action to address this issue, inadvertently misjudging the care provided.
- becoming overly sensitive fearing that if this is what happens when they are present, what happens when they leave.

Regular family members need to be supported by understanding the behaviors of their family member as well as the behaviors of others around them. The more they are equipped to manage the behaviors, the more comfortable our setting and the more they are willing to visit.

c) Relationships:

Mentally Impaired Male Client
with a Mentally Impaired Female Client

At times a specific mentally impaired male client will be attracted to a specific mentally impaired female client, or visa versa. When a mentally impaired client always seeks out the *same* male or female client there is probably a legitimate reason. Something about that client either reminds him of his spouse or something about that client hooks an old memory from the past (a past girl friend).

Once sitting together, their sexual responsiveness may escalate. They will begin by holding hands, hugging, kissing, fondling and then exposing each. It is important to emphasize that there is no premeditated thought. The libido is stimulated and the clients respond. There is no way to keep the two apart unless they are heavily medicated, physically restrained or re-located. None of these interventions are desirable.

The need for sexual intimacy is natural and with the dementia client may only intensify due to their loneliness and fear. On one unit, it was common to find a male and female dementia client sitting on the couch together, the female client fast asleep with her head on the shoulder of the male client. The male client sitting with a wide grin and obviously content with the arrangement.

Unfortunately, caregivers with restricted ideation around sexual behavior will probably want to intervene because of the consequences of prolonged contact - fondling and exposing each other. Intervention on this behavior should only occur if:

one of the clients is distressed by the contact of the other
or
prior to their fondling or exposing each other in view of others.

The latter case requires the care team to pattern the behavior, identifying the times of day when they are usually in contact with each other and the length of time from initial contact to the point of fondling or exposing each other. The care team is then responsible to check within the time frame of initial contact and distract them apart prior to the action that negates their dignity.

A problem can arise when the spouse of one of the client's is still alive. In this case, the visiting spouse must be helped to understand the behavior - taught that their spouse is probably no longer aware of being married and the relationship stems from an association with someone in his past life. This will not always be acceptable to the visiting spouse. Even knowing the rationale behind his actions, she may find it difficult to remain objective when she sees her husband sitting with another woman and holding hands.

In the case where the wife cannot handle what is happening, the care team must then take the initiative to decrease the stress created by the situation. She must be encouraged to call the unit a half hour before each visit or set a regular visiting time, and instruct other family members to do the same. In that way the care team can then separate the two clients before the visit, having one occupied with an activity while the wife is visiting.

This is the same intervention that family would be encouraged to take if a client had a history of aggressive behavior. Family would be asked to call before each visit to ensure that it is a "good time." There is no difference in this case. The behavior is beyond the control of the client and therefore must be controlled by the care team.

d) Relationships:

A Cognitively Well Male Client
with a Mentally Impaired Female Client

The circumstances of this situation will dictate the response.

> If a cognitively well male client is known to be a very caring and trustworthy gentleman, who initially began a supportive friendship with a level two mentally impaired female client that turned into an intimate relationship, would you intervene?

If the mentally impaired client responds in a positive manner, it is hoped that no one would intervene. There are no bounds to loving someone. If there were, then a number of existing relationships between well and frail individuals would be in jeopardy. The key here is that the relationship grew to intimacy and the mentally impaired client was responding to that person's affection in a positive manner.

In the same vein, it is necessary to discuss another delicate issue. Sometimes a cognitively well male client may target mentally impaired female clients, fondling or exposing them. In this situation, the attending physician must be asked if the male client would be considered <u>mentally incompetent</u>. If the answer is *no*, then the response is obvious. This behavior would not be accepted anywhere else. If in the community a person took advantage of someone who was mentally incompetent, he would be charged with sexual assault *regardless of his age*.

A long term care facility has no freedom to have any different expectations. If this situation should arise, then the cognitively well client must be warned that his behavior has serious legal ramifications. He must be counseled to assist in stopping his behavior. If it continues, he must be charged. Some may believe that such an intervention is harsh and unrealistic because the client is "old." On the contrary, to treat the situation any differently is in contrast to our philosophy of care. We are responsible for the physical well being and safety of those under our care. Secondly, to protect a cognitively well client just because he is "old" is a stereotypic expectation that the courts would not accept and we cannot tolerate (see ageism in the text Breaking Through: Working with the Frail Elderly).

e) Relationships:

Mentally Impaired Male Client
with a Mentally Impaired Male Client

Mentally Impaired Female Client
with a Mentally Impaired Female Client

Homosexuality is acceptable within our society. The sexual orientation of an individual will not change simply because the person develops dementia. Two primary issues arise with homosexual behavior by dementia clients:

- when the partner a homosexual dementia client chooses is heterosexual and becomes distressed or aggressive by any of his/her advances.

- if caregivers, family members, visitors and cognitively well clients are challenged by heterosexual behavior they will face an even greater challenge with homosexual behavior.

Homosexual behavior will need a skilled care team to address the conflicts that may arise between clients and an effective education and support mechanism to ensure objectivity by all stakeholders.

Part Two: Causes of Sexually Expressive Behavior

An overview of the potential causes for sexual expressive behavior include:

> Medication
> Depression
> Sensory Deprivation
> False Cueing
> Bored
> Urinary Tract Infection
> Physical Intimacy
> Old Behavior
> Control
> Timing
> Misinterpretation of Person
> Misinterpretation of Place
> Rapport
> Culture
> Physical Need/Discomfort

It is important to emphasize that much of the discussion on sexual behavior will involve the male client. Although the sexual behavior of the female client does present some challenges, sexual behavior of the male client towards female caregivers or female clients is more likely to spark greater concerns. This can be demonstrated quite easily.

- A female dementia client who pats the bottom of male or female caregivers is often considered 'cute' by members of the care team. However, a male dementia client demonstrating the same behavior will usually be seen in a different light.

- A female client hugging a female caregiver can have a different impact than a male client hugging that same caregiver.

It is the actions of the male dementia client who seems to stir the greatest challenges.

Medication
Many medications will have a direct impact on sexual behavior, i.e. some psychotropic medications create prolonged erections. However, it is anti-depressive medication that will often cause sexual expressive behavior with the dementia client. The following discussion on depression will define the relationship between anti-depressive medication and sexual behavior.

Depression
Research has identified that 75% or more of those with dementia experience depression. The mentally impaired may not know exactly what they have lost, but they have a constant foreboding that something is missing, hence the depressive response.

The common experience of depression is loneliness. Although the need to resolve this loneliness can be intense, the ability to satisfy that need depends on the degree of apathy and amount of energy available. Viewing depression as a trough will demonstrate the behavioral shifts that will occur.

The diagram demonstrates how a person can move through a depressive cycle. There are three points in the depressive cycle - going into depression (point 1), deep depression (point 2) and coming out of depression (point 3). During deep depression or the bottom of the trough (point 2), the individual

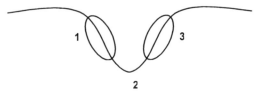

experiences significant apathy and low energy (the common symptoms of depression). During this time the person does not have the energy or desire to address the intense feelings of loneliness. However, going into depression or sliding down the trough (point 1) or coming out of depression as a result of an anti-depressive medication or up the trough (point 3), the person still experiences the severe loneliness but has the energy and desire to resolve it. With the mentally impaired, going or coming out of depression will result in their grabbing and/or holding onto anyone who comes close.

Supportive Measure
1) Caregiver and Volunteer Contact - When depression is suspected or the person demonstrating sexual expressive behavior is on an anti-depressive medication then addressing the loneliness is the primary objective. Caregivers (from all departments) and volunteers comfortable with physical contact (hugging, touching and/or massaging) should be encouraged to maintain that contact with this client.

2) Pets and Children Programs - Needless to say involvement with intergenerational and pet visitation programs would assist in addressing the loneliness.

3) Massage Therapist - Registered massage therapists are an excellent resource to long term care and other health care organizations providing therapeutic relaxation message, and addressing the need for physical contact.

4) Scheduling - It is important that physical contact with this client be scheduled throughout the day (defined by the Care Plan Summary and monitored by the Programming Map). There is nothing more disheartening than to witness continual contact by a variety of individuals over a few hours and then little contact the remainder of the day. Scheduled care, departmental visits (housekeeping, dietary, etc.), volunteer visits, programming opportunities, family visits, etc. should be scheduled throughout the entire day to ensure consistent contact on an hourly basis.

Sensory Deprivation

One of the primary areas for sensory deprivation involves touch. A dementia client void of physical contact other than through care will often demonstrate sensory deprivation by touching anyone who comes near.

Supportive Measure

1) Sensory Stimulation - Sensory stimulation programs attempt to simulate all five senses - touch, smell, sight, hearing and taste. There are many examples of sensory stimulation programs (see Programming). One example is a sensory box to stimulate tactile sensation. The contents of a sensory box includes fabrics and materials with a variety of textures (sand paper, velvet, terrycloth, etc.). Emptying the contents of the sensory box on a table and allowing this client to feel each piece of material provides a variety of tactile sensations.

2) Caregiver Contact, Pet/Children Programs, Massage Therapist - as described above.

False Cueing

The term false cueing implies that the dementia client responds to a stimuli without the knowledge of his location or circumstances. A mentally impaired male client does not know that he is sick, does not know that others around him are sick, and does not know where he is. He can easily misinterpret the actions of others. When this client sits next to an individual experiencing sensory deprivation, a female client who continually touches others, he will respond to the stimuli.

Supportive Measure

1) Avoiding Contact - In this situation both clients react to each other. Neither are seeking out the other, as described earlier. The action of the male is based totally on the stimuli received. The close proximity of the male client encourages the client with sensory stimulation to touch. The male dementia client interprets the actions of the female client as an advance and responds accordingly. In this case, it is necessary to assist the male client who misinterprets the stimuli and to protect the female client who experiences the

consequences of her actions. It is the responsibility of the entire care team to monitor the male client's location. The male client needs to be directed to a chair away from the client who touches others. If he is found sitting next to this female client, he should be moved to another location.

2)   Communicating - The supportive measure to address the behavior needs to be communicated to the care team (utilizing the Care Plan Summary).

Urinary Tract Infection
It is easy to misinterpret fondling or rubbing of genitals as masturbation when in fact some clients may be experiencing burning or irritation due to a urinary tract or yeast infection.

Supportive Measures
1)   Medical History - A standard medical history should identify if there is a history of chronic urinary tract or yeast infection, and that information communicated to the care team.

2)   Medical Exam - A behavioral care practices manual (as identified in chapter one) should identify an automatic medical exam to rule out possible infection when consistent genital rubbing occurs.

Physical Intimacy
A question that must be asked of family is, "How did your family member show his/her affection in the past?" If family respond that their family member always hugged or put his arm around the shoulders of those he was close to, then the need for physical intimacy for this individual is probably high.

However, the opportunity in a health care facility to display or receive such contact is often minimal. With minimal physical contact, the need for "touch" becomes strong. The client will unconsciously compensate by frequently touching those near him. When he touches female staff or clients, he can easily be labeled by some as "a dirty old man." When labeled, some caregivers may be uncomfortable with his behavior and avoid him as much as possible. When avoided, his need for physical intimacy only intensifies. His touching increases in order to satisfy that need, which only intensifies the labeling, increasing the avoidance behavior, further increasing the need and so on.

Supportive Measure

1) Caregiver Contact - In this situation caregivers have a number of responsibilities. The first is obvious, this person has a significant need for physical contact. When in contact with this client, caregivers need to initiate touch - consciously slipping their arm over his shoulder when walking alongside him, or placing a hand over his while standing next to him. In each instance, caregivers must consistently provide the needed physical contact that is required.

Secondly, those who perceive the behavior as inappropriate may react to those caregivers making physical contact with some aversion. In one case a male client was labeled by some caregivers as a 'dirty old man' because he continually attempted to hug and touch people around him. The case was reviewed at a care conference. The client's family indicated that this male client always expressed his affection by hugging or putting his arm around others. At the end of the review, all members of the care team stated that they understood the rationale behind his behavior and agreed that their perception of him was inaccurate requiring them to address his need for physical contact.

Shortly after the care conference a staff member on maternity leave brought her new baby onto the unit. She approached this male client with her baby. As she was about to place the baby in this man's arms a caregiver who was part of the care conference shouted, "Don't give the baby to him, you don't know what he will do." The new mother was asked how she felt about the situation, her comment was, "As long as we watch, I don't think there will be a problem." The baby was placed in this man's arms, he was gentle, smiled and cooed, rocking the baby in his arms. It is not easy to change the attitudes of others. Individuals with restrictive sexual ideation often respond by reflex.

The third responsibility is to advocate on behalf of the client. Those who understand the behavior and are comfortable providing the needed physical contact cannot be swayed because of the attitudes of others.

2) Pets/Children - These are valuable programming opportunities for the individual requiring physical contact, but it will be necessary to override the resistance by those who view the client's behavior as 'sexually inappropriate'.

3) Family and Volunteer Support - Some family members and/or volunteers may need to be directed in addressing the need for physical contact. Although sitting and holding hands or having an arm around a dementia client may seem straight forward, some family members or volunteers may need encouragement to initiate such contact, as well as direction on when it should be provided, how long to make the contact and those clients who do not respond well to such contact.

Old Behavior
A question that must be asked of the spouse of a dementia male client demonstrating sexual expressive behavior is - What was your husband like when he was around other women? (adult children may not know the true answer to this question.) If she answers that he was a 'flirt', then she has provided significant insight into his present behavior.

This type of male was an opportunist when he was cognitively well, often looking for a woman who would respond to his advances. Every woman has met this male at a party. When he approaches his target his initial advances are subtle. Should the woman become offended he can easily back away implying that she misunderstood, then look for a new target until he receives the desired response. This type of behavior is well ingrained as a part of the client's pre-morbid personality. Now that he is mentally impaired in a long term care facility he has many targets (female staff, volunteers, family visitors and other clients), however his loss of cognitive ability and inhibition means that he is no longer subtle. He is now very descriptive in his language and direct in his actions regardless of the location or who is present.

Supportive Measure

1) Old Response - When a behavior is linked to a client's pre-morbid personality, then it is important to discover from family how they responded to that behavior in the past. In the case where a male client was a flirt in the past, the wife must be asked what she said or did when her husband was flirtatious and she wanted to stop him. If she answers, "I just said John, woman do not like that, please stop.", then the old response may still retain the desired results.

2) Patterning - Patterning this behavior is valuable. A time pattern may not be present, however there is usually an event pattern. The event pattern often reveals that a certain location (i.e. the lounge) or circumstances (i.e. group activity) is where his behavior is the most intense. The care team will have to be vigilant when he is in these locations or during these events, defining the pre-emptive cues that indicate his behavioral response, then distracting him from his target.

Control

Part of a client's history should also uncover the past marital relationship. The adult children are usually a more accurate source for this information. Often when the spouse is asked to describe her relationship with her husband, she will probably respond "It was fine." However if the adult children are asked about the relationship between their parents they would probably respond that their mother was controlled by their father, where she made few decisions and was treated with little respect.

The ability of a husband to treat his wife in this manner may reflect his perception of women in general. In the past, this individual's attitudes may have been camouflaged, although he treated his wife as though she were chattel and degraded women in a vulgar manner with his "buddies", he was probably very guarded in his comments or actions towards women directly. His present loss of inhibition means that his comments, gestures and mannerisms are expressed freely with any woman he encounters.

Supportive Measure

1) Stand Firm - Street smart caregivers will often respond well to this client's sexually expressive language and mannerisms (revealed

through the 24 Hour Profile, see assessment). They stand firm, remain objective and issue a simple command, "John please stop what you are doing." Caregivers with less experience become flustered and seem to only intensify his response. Caregivers who struggle with this behavior require training and support in how to control their emotions and reactions with clients who are sexually intimidating.

2) Providing Control - This client needs the feeling that he is in control. Although he is mentally impaired, he usually does not respond well to female caregivers who tell him what he should do. His sexually explicit language only intensifies when he is pressured by a female caregiver. Providing him with the feeling that he is making the decisions regarding his care or programs will often decrease the intensity of his behavior.

3) Safeguarding Other Clients - The female dementia client living on a unit who believes she works there is vulnerable around this individual. This is the dementia client who attempts to take care of other clients or tells them where they should be or what they should be doing. Unfortunately she does not know to avoid this male client, she cannot remember his outbursts from the last contact and is unable to read the cues indicating that he does not tolerate what she is doing. Likewise, this male dementia client does not know the female is mentally impaired, only that she is continually pressuring him. The time pattern of the female client attempting to care for others on the unit must be defined and her behavior redirected away from this male client or the male client moved to a different location when she is busy caring for others (see Programming Focus).

Timing
Timing represents the client's energy level at different times of the day. The peak for physical and mental energy creates different behavioral dynamics. Some dementia clients will become sexually aroused if intimate care (such as bathing or peri-care) is scheduled in the morning, but not aroused if it is scheduled in the evening. In the morning clients are generally at their peak of physical energy, having the physical ability to become aroused. In the evening they are physically tired and less able to become aroused.

Others may become sexually aroused when intimate tasks are scheduled during the evening but not aroused if scheduled in the morning. This now involves mental energy. The client's mental ability is generally highest when the client is well rested, allowing the client to be less influenced by the stimuli. However as the dementia client becomes tired, confusion is increased, resulting in the stimuli being misinterpreted causing sexual arousal.

Supportive Measure
1) Trial and Error Assessment - When a dementia client becomes aroused as a result of intimate care during a certain time of the day, then an alternate time should be scheduled to see if the response is lessened.

Bored
Boredom is a common problem for many dementia clients. A dementia client could sit for extended periods unless something is scheduled for the person or contact is made by someone. When bored, many dementia clients will usually find something to do. Physically touching others, masturbation, undressing, etc. can be a response to inactivity.

Supportive Measure
1) Patterning - Boredom is a common reason for many behaviors. It is important to define the time pattern of the behavior in order to best schedule programming. Programming should then be scheduled in advance of the behavior.

2) Programming - There are a variety of programming opportunities for the dementia client regardless of the individual's functioning ability (see section on Programming and Programming Map).

Misinterpretation of Person
Much to the chagrin of many caregivers, they inadvertently stimulate sexual expressive behavior by the dementia client. In long term care or any health care facility, a dementia client does not know where he is, that he is sick or that the person performing the care is a caregiver. The client responds to intimate contact by a female caregiver (during

peri-care, undressing or bathing) as any male would respond to such contact by a female. It is natural for a male to become aroused when being undressed or touched intimately by a woman.

<u>Supportive Measures</u>
1) Stop the Stimuli - Those uncomfortable with this behavior will often complain that the client is having an erection and still attempt to complete the bath or peri-care. Persistent contact at this time can escalate the behavior to sexual aggression. When a client becomes sexually aroused during intimate care, stop the contact for a few moments to allow the client to settle, and then resume the care task.

2) Do Not Overreact - The caregiver's reaction to the client's sexual arousal must be neutral or indifferent. The dementia male client is usually not aware of being aroused. Any comments or actions by the caregiver may confuse the client and result in an aggressive response.

3) Male Presence - Having a male caregiver complete intimate care will usually eliminate sexual expressive behavior. However, there are few male caregivers in the health care profession. Having a male manager, housekeeper or maintenance man present during certain intimate tasks seems to decrease arousal. The male manager, housekeeper or maintenance man would not be involved in the care. They would simply stand in sight of the client carrying on a conversation. The presence of a male seems to distract the client while the female caregiver is performing the care. Of course confidentiality, privacy issues and the comfort level of the male providing the support, as well as the client's reaction to the presence of the male support must always be considered.

4) Diversional Measures - Music or client specific conversation (something that relates to the client's past history) will often distract the client during intimate care tasks, decreasing the tendency to become aroused.

Misinterpretation of Place
A dementia client living in a health care facility does not know where he is and that the people around him are also mentally impaired.

Bedroom doors left open while clients are undressing; bathroom doors open while clients are on the toilet; and even some clients walking down the hall naked can be a common experience on some units. As a result, this stimuli can be sexually stimulating to the male dementia client.

Supportive Measure
1) Patterning - This behavior demonstrates a specific time pattern. It usually occurs late morning and is rarely seen at any other time of the day. What stimulates the client is the concentrated morning care regime common on many units. When the time pattern reveals that the client is sexually expressive during late morning, then supportive measures (i.e. programming) are required by mid morning to remove the client from the stimuli.

2) Programming - Removing the client from the stimuli (called a retracting measure) will decrease his arousal and subsequent sexual behavior. Family or volunteer visits at this time, or involvement in a recreation program off the unit will achieve the desired results.

3) Care Practices - On some units there are times when caregivers need to be reminded about client privacy and dignity. If bathroom doors hamper effective positioning or safe access then they should be removed and replaced with a privacy curtain. Privacy curtains are unobtrusive and still hide the bathroom from view of others. It is always important to adapt the environment to the care needs of the clientele being served.

Rapport
A female dementia client on one unit would always pat the bottom of anyone she appeared to like. Many caregivers considered her behavior as cute. However a male dementia client maintaining the same behavior can be labeled by some as a 'dirty old man.' This duality in interpretation often results in conflict between caregivers - those who accept the behavior only when it is demonstrated by a female client, versus those who accept the behavior regardless of who demonstrates it.

Supportive Measures
1) Staff Education - Unless caregivers receive formal education and support on sexual expressive behavior there will always be this dichotomy of approach and attitude within the care team.

2) Client Advocacy - The caregiver who objectively interprets the behavior of a client must defend the client regardless of the comments or perceptions of those less tolerant of that behavior. A Client Advocate Program is a formal mechanism that defines specific caregivers to represent a client during any discussion. The role of the advocate is to challenge those who misinterpret the behavior and resist any actions that are not in the best interest of the client.

3) Accountability - Caregivers who persist in judging a client's behavior and alter their contact as a result must be held accountable for their actions. When education, caregiver supports and care mechanisms are developed to maintain the individuality of the client, and despite these initiatives certain caregivers still impose their personal assessment of the situation it must be considered as direct insubordination. No client advocacy program nor care practice will ever be totally effective unless accountability within the organization is a common practice.

4) Communication - To prevent misjudging what is occurring and ensure the appropriate response when encountered, managers, part time and full time staff of all departments, regular family visitors and volunteers, must be informed of the rationale behind this client's behavior (see Care Plan Summary).

5) Visitor or Family Information Package - Family and volunteers require information on ways dementia clients communicate rapport i.e. touching, hugging, patting bottoms, etc. Providing information in advance will assist them to be prepared for what they may encounter.

Culture
Italians are well known for their warm and exuberant welcome when someone enters their home (as are other cultures). An Italian mentally impaired client lived on a secured dementia special needs unit (see

Modular Care) and thought the unit was his home. He would frequently wait by the entrance door to the unit. When anyone entered the unit he would greet them with a hug and a kiss, and then escort them to the nursing station. Visitors to the unit would eventually expect his welcome after encountering this man a few times. However new visitors to the unit were not prepared for his greeting and would pull away when he tried to make contact. Their pulling away only intensified the client's behavior and could eventually result in an aggressive response should they not accept his greeting.

Supportive Measures
1) Warning about Greeters - Many units housing dementia clients have some type of greeter. Individuals not familiar with the unit or these individuals will often respond in a manner that will only intensify the behavior or result in an aggressive response. The unit housing the Italian gentleman addressed the issue by placing a sign on the entrance door preparing visitors for his contact. The sign said "You may be greeted by Luigi, a friendly gentleman who will escort you to the nursing station." This provided warning of what awaited on the other side of the door and allowed visitors to respond accordingly.

2) Information Package and Orientation Session - The volunteer, family and new staff information packages and orientation sessions must alert these individuals to greeters, the variety of greetings they may encounter and how to respond when experienced.

Physical Need or Discomfort
Any physical need or discomfort can result in a dementia client demonstrating what can be considered sexual expressive behavior - exposing herself, rubbing genitals, etc.

- When a dementia client becomes too warm, she will take her clothes off.
- If uncomfortable with what he is wearing, he will remove it.
- Needs to go to the bathroom, he will undress and go.
- Has an itch or discomfort in her genitalia, she will scratch it.
- Believes it is time for bed, he will undress.

The loss of inhibition results in any physical discomfort or need being addressed regardless of the location or who is around.

Supportive Measures

1) Investigate the Cause - A client who continually removes his/her clothes is often communicating a need not related to sexual behavior. In one case a client gained weight after admission but was still wearing her original clothes. When the tight fitting clothing made her uncomfortable she removed it. Once the clothing was altered and new clothing of a proper size purchased the behavior was eliminated. It is often valuable to investigate the simplest things before looking for a more complex cause, i.e. removing an itchy sweater before the client removes it.

2) Patterning - Defining the time and event pattern will provide direction on what is creating the behavior and when it should be addressed i.e. undressing when the curtains are drawn, because the client may believe it is time for bed. Behavior communicates. Patterning will assist to identify what the client is trying to tell us.

Chapter Ten

Admission

Imagine the following:

I approach you
Place a blindfold over your eyes,
Plug your ears so you cannot hear./
I take you to an unknown destination
Telling you nothing of where you are going or why./

I remove your blindfold and ear plugs.
You find yourself in an unfamiliar building./
In a large crowded room with people you have never seen before./
I leave with instructions to those in the room
Not to let you through any of the doors to the outside./

You can find nothing in the room to help you identify your
     location./
The people who confront you speak a language you have never
     heard before./
You find yourself unable to decipher any meaning from their
     attempts to communicate with you./

People are constantly moving about.
Some are touching your clothing
Placing you here, then there./
Even when you refuse to follow, they take you./
Your attempts to leave the building are always thwarted.
At times their behavior seems quite bizarre and threatening./

It is getting dark.
You believe your family should be missing you by now and
    coming to get you.
Instead you are taken to a bedroom with two beds in it./
A person lies motionless in the bed by the door.
No sound, no reaction to the activities around./
You are stripped of your clothing.
Then dressed in a funny shirt backwards.
And motioned to lie down on the empty bed./
The lights are turned out./

You cannot rest.
You hear unfamiliar noises from outside the door./
Periodically in the darkness a figure walks into the room with a
    flashlight.
It is shone in your direction.
Then the person leaves./

The sun rises./
Someone comes to you,
Hands you a bowl with water and two pieces of cloth./
You do not understand what is asked./
The individual takes the cloth, places it in the water
And then moves the cloth to your face.
You attempt to stop her, but are unsuccessful./

You never know where you are./
Who the people are around you.
Faces and things never remain constant./
The fear you experience never leaves you./
Each day the experience is the same./

That scenario closely portrays the experience of a mentally impaired
individual being admitted to a long term care facility or a hospital.

The Difference

It is important to differentiate the experiences of a cognitively well older client admitted to health care facility from those with dementia. A person who is cognitively well can be prepared and supported through the entire admission process.

- Admission is usually discussed with that person well in advance.
- There is an opportunity for the cognitively well to:
  - express their concerns and fears.
  - clarify issues that are not understood.
  - visit the facility in advance and familiarize herself with the surroundings.
  - meet some of the staff that may be performing her care.
- On the day of admission she can:
  - be supported by other clients, staff and family.
  - be re-familiarized with the surroundings by touring the unit again.
  - be given written instructions and routines left to help remember what must be done and when.
  - have the opportunity to talk to others as needed about her fears, and helped as often as needed with the transition.

There are no such luxuries in preparing the mentally impaired individual for admission.

- No matter what is said prior to that day, it will be forgotten.
- No matter what is discussed on the way to the facility, it will be forgotten.
- No matter what steps are taken to orientate this person to the people and surroundings, they will be forgotten.

All that will be experienced is a bombarding of stimuli in a very short period of time, causing intense confusion to what is happening.

As will be discussed, admission to a health care facility is a complex process that must be well planned. Without doing so, considerable turmoil will be experienced by the newly admitted, mentally impaired individual, their family and the staff involved.

In long term care, the first week of admission is a crucial period for many new clients who are mentally impaired. That period can be a time where this person establishes either a state of security or one of intense fear. Within the first few days of arriving on the unit, a new admission with limited mental ability is expected to respond appropriately to:

- a bath given by someone who is not familiar, in an environment that is unknown.
- sleep the first few nights in a room that now has one or more roommates who are not known, and whose behavior may not be understood.
- eat in a dining room where twenty to thirty other people are eating, where noise and movement is constant.
- function in a setting that has a maze of rooms.
- unfamiliar people performing intimate care tasks, whose faces change every eight hours.

If this is the case, then the expectations are in error.

The mentally impaired are admitted to long term care for one very specific reason - they can no longer cope living in homes they have known for years, with a spouse or family around who they have associated with most of their lives. For the mentally impaired, the first few days of admission can only create a feeling of helplessness and an elevation of anxiety. In that state of emotional saturation, mental functioning is decreased. Simple tasks that were easily done the day before will be temporarily lost upon entering the facility. The behavioral responses can be varied and mixed - wandering, elopement, calling out, crying, aggression, etc.

Admission to any health care facility by a mentally impaired client can be referred to as Transition Shock:

A period of time where the person experiences dramatic change
in a short period causing abilities to decrease and
their level of dysfunctioning to increase.

This is well supported by the frequent comments by the family of a new admission. They will often state shortly after admitting their loved one to the facility, "I never realized that my mother was so confused." What they are witnessing is mother's response to dramatic change.

The first experiences of a new admission could dictate his response to that unit for an extended period of time. If within the first week there is a constant sense of panic, the emotional distress and fear in some may last for a considerable period of time. It could easily take a month for a newly admitted mentally impaired client to gain any familiarity to the smallest aspects of the unit, the care and the people performing it. In fact, the panic level initiated during the first few days of admission could take considerably longer to subside, and for some, it may never be lessened.

This is not to imply that making the admission process more sensitive to the needs of the mentally impaired will eliminate all aggressive and wandering behavior of new clients. As we have stated, there is no one supportive measure that will put an end to all of the symptoms experienced by the mentally impaired. A supportive admission process does lessen the dramatic behavioral swings encountered, making admission a more tolerable experience for the client who must live through it, for the family who must witness it and for the staff who are required to cope with it.

The responsibility of the unit is to make that first week of admission a process of gradual change. The steps taken at that time will decrease the upheaval and problems encountered. To discuss these steps, we need to divide the admission process into three areas:

1) Introductory Period
2) Transition Period
3) Orientation Period

It is important to emphasize that not all facilities will be able to incorporate all aspects of these strategies. The challenge facing the facility is to determine which are achievable and then define alternate ways to achieve similar outcomes when not available.

1) The Introductory Period

The Introductory Period is the time before admission. Knowing this client cannot be prepared for admission in advance, this period of time allows the care team and family an opportunity to prepare. This is when the new client and his family are required to make contact in advance with the unit and the staff who will possibly provide the care. It also allows members of the care team the opportunity to meet this client before admission to gain some critical information that cannot be easily obtained by any pre-assessment forms.

a)   Pre-admission Meeting

Pre-admission meetings of perspective clients are not new for most facilities. What varies is the timing of those meetings. Some will meet the family and possibly the perspective resident months before possible admission, while others will meet them only days or hours in advance.

Unfortunately, many facilities limit that meeting to only a select few participants from the facility. The pre-admission meeting must not only include the charge nurse (unit manager) of the unit where this new admission will most likely be placed, but also a direct line representative of that care team. The goal of this contact is to establish some direction on what needs to be done or not done during the first few days of admission. It also provides an opportunity for the client and his family to meet someone who will possibly be providing that care.

If the new client is in hospital prior to admission and unable to attend the pre-admission meeting, it is important that the charge nurse and/or staff member from the unit have the opportunity to visit the potential client in that setting. This will allow staff the opportunity to talk personally with hospital personnel who have performed much of this individual's care. This meeting provides the chance to identify what has already been found successful and what should be avoided.

The pre-admission meeting provides staff the opportunity to ask specific questions regarding issues that are very relevant to their day-to-day care routines. In the event that a face-to-face pre-admission meeting cannot be arranged, then a phone meeting with the family or an e-mail contact (if available) is still valuable. Arranging a phone meeting, where the discussion is on speaker, allows more than one member of the care team to hear the responses and ask the necessary questions.

b) Pre-admission Assessment

Direct line staff need more specific information from the family caregiver than what is normally provided by most pre-admission assessment forms. Knowing that this person is incontinent is not enough. The caregiver needs to ask, "How do you know when your mother has to go to the bathroom?" Likewise, uncovering that the new client resists taking medication does not solve the challenges facing that task. Staff would need to ask, "Which jam does your mother like to eat?" which allows the opportunity to successfully camouflage the prescribed drugs. Detailed information such as this is essential for staff in the first few days of admission.

If this information is not gained before admission, there is no question that it will be discovered days after admission. Through trial and error, staff in that first few weeks or months will invariably learn what they must do or not do. Unfortunately, discovering the information after admission is not only a waste of time and energy, but it comes at the expense of the new admission. Without having an opportunity to gain the individualized data prior to admission, the care team is unable to respond specifically to this person's needs, thus resulting in major behavioral swings that are difficult to control.

The following identifies much of the information required on a new admission and comprises an excellent Family Questionnaire.

Meals:
Likes and dislikes?
What will your relative eat if everything else is refused?
What will your relative never eat?
When is your relative's main meal?
What are normal meal times?
How much does your relative eat at each meal?
What problems have you had getting your relative to eat?
Any special arrangements or utensils used during meal time?
Does your relative snack during the day (if yes, what and when)?

Dressing:
What can your relative do regarding dressing and undressing?
What does your relative need help with?
Do you have any problems dressing or undressing your relative?
　　- if yes, what and how do you deal with it?
Is there anything your relative enjoys wearing more than others?

Toileting:
How do you know when your relative has to go to the bathroom?
Is your relative incontinent?
　　- if so, how cooperative is your relative when being changed?
Is there a pattern, special times or a manner that helps with
　　toileting?
Are there any medications or foods taken to assist with your
　　relative's bowels?

Bathing:
Does your relative normally have a bath or shower?
What time of day?
Any problems in bathing?
Any special precautions or arrangements?
Would you be willing to be present during your relative's first
　　bath or two after admission?

Grooming:

Problems combing and washing hair?

Problems with mouth care?

Does your relative brush his/her own teeth or do you do it for him/her?

If your relative wears glasses, when does he/she wear them?

Ambulation:

Does your relative wander?

- if yes, when and how long?

Are there any concerns about your relative's ability to walk?

When are your relative's rest times?

What type of shoes does your relative wear?

Does your relative use any walking aids - cane, railing, walker, etc.?

Activities:

What activities have you found your relative enjoys now?

What activities did your relative do in the past that are not done now?

How long can your relative participate in an activity?

What is the best time for your relative to do activities?

Do you take your relative on outings?

- if yes, where, when and how long?

What do you talk about?

What topics of conversation upset your relative and should be avoided?

Does your relative watch TV or listen to music?

- if yes, what type and when?

How often do you plan to visit and for how long?

Who else from your family plans to visit?

Are you willing to assist with activities or outings?

- if yes, which day and time is most convenient?

Sleeping:

What time does your relative normally go to bed?

Is your relative up during the night?
- if yes, how often?
- what occurs when your relative is up?
- how do you get your relative back to bed?
- what is your relative's mental state during that time?
Does your relative sleep during the day?
- if yes, when & how long?
Anything special about your relatives bed or room (personal quilt, number of pillows, light on, etc.)?

Normal Day:
Describe a normal day for your relative.
When are your relative's "bad times" of the day?
How do you deal with those times?
How would we know that your relative is getting anxious or agitated?
Do you have any problems getting your relative to take medication?
Any special preparations for taking medications?
What things does your relative find comforting?
How does your relative relate to new people?

Understanding Your Relative:
Describe your relative twenty years ago.
How has your relative dealt with stress in the past?
Knowing that past memory influences present behavior, what past event(s) (positive and negative) stand out in your relative's life?

These questions need to be provided to the family in written form prior to admission with instructions to complete as much as possible in advance of the admission day. The questionnaire can then be reviewed on admission day (see following section).

c) Admission Time

The time of day of any admission must be set by the care team. Admission should be at a time when the unit is experiencing the least amount of activity. When the unit is at a low activity level it decreases the amount of bombarding stimuli this new client is subjected to during the first few hours on the unit. That alone will have a significant calming effect on this person's fear level. You can imagine the results if this new admission is first introduced to the unit at its most chaotic time. There is nothing more frustrating than to see a mentally impaired individual admitted in the morning when the care team is engulfed in the routines of the unit, and little attention can be given to him or his family during those first few trying hours. Admission time must occur when staff can realistically focus their attention on this person.

d) Personal Belongings

It is also important at the pre-admission meeting or contact to identify with family the personal articles of the new admission that they intend to bring in and how they should be arranged in that person's room. These details need to be discussed in advance of admission and family instructed that these articles arrive a few hours before admission.

Having the person's articles arrive at the same time that he is admitted is of little value. Usually the articles are whisked away to be labelled and the person does not get them until later that day or even the next day. Familiar articles must be in place <u>before</u> the client walks onto the unit. In this way, the new client sees a room that already has a degree of familiarity attached to it, decreasing much of the transition anxiety by eliminating some of the foreign element.

e) Preparing for the Day

The pre-admission meeting also allows the care team to establish with family:

- what meal the new client would best relate to on the first day and if family are prepared to have three servings of that meal

delivered from a local restaurant at admission time if the dietary department cannot supply it.
- the appropriate activity (something the new client is used to doing) the family, new client and staff can be involved in for the first afternoon.
- what the client likes to talk about.
- what topics should be avoided.

The more information that can be obtained to plan that first day, the more effective the care team will be in decreasing the transition shock felt by the client. This information is an integral part of the admission day (see next section).

f) Involvement on the First Day
Sometimes family feel that it is best to just drop their family member off at the facility and leave soon after. On the contrary, it must be stressed with family that their participation in settling their family member on that day is crucial to the admission process.

New families will not know the busy or slack times during the shift. The care team must identify for family the best and worst times for them to leave the unit on that first day. It is important for staff to outline their normal schedule for that shift and the next. Family need to be instructed that they cannot leave between:

- 1445 hours and 1515 hours if the staff shift change is at 1500 hours.
- 1630 hours and 1730 hours if half the staff are at their supper and the other half are serving the clients supper.

For family to leave during the times when caregivers know they are not available does not allow anyone to support their relative.

g) Pre-Visits
Pre-visits can be arranged prior to admission. This can be during the day, evening or on weekends, whichever time is best for family. The

pre-visit provides an opportunity to bring the potential client in a few days prior to admission for a meal, or to attend a specific function.

Advance contact with the unit will give the care team and family an indication of some of the problems that may be experienced on admission day. Mother's reaction to the environment, the stimuli, other clients, the activities, etc. can be noted and plans made in advance outlining how to deal with those issues on the upcoming day.

It is important that family be part of this process in order to decrease their fears about the facility and define their role in this client's care. The more this can be achieved in advance, the more apt families are to remain an integral part of this client's life after admission.

2) The Transition Period

a) Care Team Support

The transition period is the first few days when the new client is admitted. During the first few hours when that new client is on the unit, it is important that a caregiver be relieved from other duties in order that she may be solely assigned to this new individual and his family. That suggestion usually raises the eyebrows of managers and staff from some facilities.

To accomplish this, it is not necessary for the facility to call in an extra staff member for an added eight hour shift, or to leave the unit short staffed. It only requires adding a four hour casual shift at the time of admission. This casual worker is to relieve a full time caregiver from her duties, allowing the regular caregiver the added time to spend with the new client.

A frequent comment to such a suggestion is that the budget does not allow for this additional cost. We need to examine this further before this option is negated on the grounds of cost. First, it is important to identify the number of yearly admissions of mentally impaired individuals at level two functioning level.

The number of admissions of level two clients to a standard sized facility would usually average two each month. Remember, that is an average. Some months it may be more and other months less. Also remember, that this number does not include new admissions representing other levels of functioning and other abilities. The need for additional staff is not necessary when admitting individuals at levels one and three of mental functioning, and those who are cognitively well/physically disabled.

Two admissions per month of level two clients translates into twenty-four half shifts per year, or a total of twelve full shifts. If converted to hours paid at a pay rate of $13.00 per hour (personal care worker) that translates to a yearly cost of $1248.00. That is a minuscule amount of any budget. The benefits of such an investment far outweigh the minimal costs. Unfortunately, even that amount will be resisted by management in some facilities who don't understand the need for such support or manage by a "nickel/dime" mentality. They look only to immediate costs, rather than the actual investment of worker hours if the support is not provided.

b) Caregiver Responsibilities

The caregiver assigned to this new client for the first shift is encouraged to spend time on an informal and formal basis with the family and new client. There are three assessment periods that must be scheduled:

1) Time where family, the new client and the caregiver are together to assess the new client's response to new people and the unit.

2) Time where the family are pre-occupied with the family questionnaire (see section on assessment), and the caregiver and new client are left alone. This is an opportunity to assess the new client's response to being without the family member's support.

3) A time where the caregiver and family discuss the family questionnaire and leave the new client alone. This allows time

to assess the response of the new client to the unit when minimal support is available.

Each of these periods needs to be expanded.

One of the easiest ways to provide the new client familiarity with the caregiver assigned, and also to decrease some of the anxiety experienced by the family, is to sit down to a pre-arranged meal. During the pre-admission meeting, family were asked which food the new client would most likely eat without much coaxing. That is what is required now.

A common question by staff to such a suggestion is, "What if the meal mother will eat is chicken, but chicken is not scheduled for the day of admission?" Many families are willing to make admission as bearable as possible. When they learn the meal may assist in the transition, they are usually willing to bring it from home, or pay to have it delivered from a nearby restaurant. Knowing that such an investment of time or money is important to help family member adapt more effectively to the transition is often enough motivation.

There is no dispute that some new admissions will not have family available to provide such support, or at some point family may refuse such a responsibility.

It is better to deal with the exceptions as they arise
and have the supports in place,
rather than to eliminate the supports
because there may be exceptions.

If family are not given direction on what they can do to help, then it is not known whether they will or not. Commonly, providing the first meal is an excellent opportunity for family to decrease much of the guilt that is experienced about placing mother in a long term care facility.

This meal must be in a room that is free from other stimuli - a location where there is a fair bit of certainty that other clients will not be milling around (remember, keep the stimuli to a minimum). That location can be an activity room or a small lounge not in use, or the dining room after everyone else has finished lunch and the room has been vacated.

During the first four hours, an opportunity should be provided for the client and caregiver to be alone, and also a time where the client is left by himself, assessing this person's response to each new situation and event. The goal is to gain as much information as quickly as possible to identify the supportive measures needed by the new admission.

Knowing in advance what will occupy the new client's time and what the person can easily talk about (identified at the pre-admission meeting) is important. Each of these can be employed to enhance rapport with the new client, decreasing that person's anxiety. More importantly, they become important supportive measures to deal with the time when the family leave the unit. There is nothing worse than having the new admission watch their family walk through the unit door. Diverting the new client's attention from the family exiting is important to prevent potential immediate behavioral changes.

c) Tapping the Family

Family members who have cared for this client prior to admission become the greatest resource in giving the care team direction and insight into the new admission's routine. If they have cared for their parent, or had significant contact with him during the progression of the disease, then they have already tested what works and what doesn't regarding approach, activities, etc. Tapping into this information is essential to prevent the care team from covering the same ground and repeating the same mistakes family may have already encountered.

It is during admission that family can be asked to complete the Family Questionnaire (identified earlier). While family are completing the questionnaire, staff have an opportunity to assess how well the new admission copes with them not present.

d) Contact with Family

The client's response to being left alone on the unit needs to be tested while family are still available. In this way, if the client is seriously distressed, family are present to assist in calming him. Then the caregiver, with the family's help, can discuss what strategies can be taken when family finally do walk away.

The caregiver's time alone with family allows the opportunity to clarify the information package provided at the pre-admission meeting. Staff can detail and answer any questions family may have on:

- their role within the facility.
- how they can be involved in the care and activities of their parent.
- communication channels that can be taken if problems are encountered.
- philosophy of the care and unit routines.

This time is needed, knowing that family members are usually inundated with information and concerns prior to admission. Likewise, this meeting will allow the caregiver to review the admission package to clarify misunderstandings.

At the end of the transition period (the first four hours), the caregiver assigned to the new admission can now formulate a basic outline of what needs to be done, how to approach this client, areas of concern, etc., and provide a specific report to the staff on duty the next shift.

3) Admission - The Orientation Period

The orientation period is the first three days after admission.

a) Caregiver Assignment
Assigning caregivers to this client for the first three days must be well planned. The goal during this period to have the least number of caregivers involved with this client and to gain as much specific information as possible. To achieve this, the caregivers assigned to

the new client on admission day must be ones who are scheduled to work the next three days.

For example: The caregiver assigned to the new admission during the first four hours, must be on duty for the next three day shifts. Likewise, the caregiver assigned to this client over the evening and night shifts must also be on duty the same shifts for the next three days. Determining who is assigned to the new admission is based solely on the rotation schedule for those days.

Once the assignment is established, a thorough assessment and communication process can be defined. The caregiver who greeted the client on the day shift, is required to report what she has uncovered about this client to the person assigned on the afternoon shift. Using that information, the caregiver is then able to maintain some consistency in approach and expectations from the guidelines established by the initial contact.

The afternoon caregiver then reports all of the information that has been gained in the last twelve hours to a specific staff member on the night shift (a summary of the four hours spent by the day person, plus her assessment of the past eight hours). The night person then reports what has occurred over the past sixteen hours to the returning day staff member. This reporting pattern occurs for three days.

The benefits of such consistency for the first three days are obvious.

- It provides the new client a degree of familiarity with caregivers assigned to perform care.
- It also provides three caregivers the opportunity to collaborate the information obtained during each shift.
- Caregivers are then able to quickly determine this client's immediate needs, strengths and limitations, and establish a baseline care plan for subsequent staff who will follow.
- Caregivers now have the most accurate direction that can be obtained in the shortest period of time.

b)   Introduction to the Care Routine

For the first three days after admission and possibly up to the first seven days, it is important that only the basics in care be completed. The care team needs to expect that this client will not respond positively to the first bath, eating in the dining room the first few meals, or sleeping the first few nights. Their responsibility to this new client during that first week of admission is to help this person gain a degree of familiarity with the unit and its staff, before feeling any pressure to perform complicated and threatening tasks.

There is no question that there will be exceptions. There are *always* exceptions to every approach or program established for the mentally impaired. It is possible that family of a new admission have been unable to perform the bath prior to entry to the unit, resulting in the new client having obvious problems with hygiene or odor that must be rectified. The care team has no choice but to initiate a bath possibly on the first day. That bath will create significant distress for the new client, potentially causing aggressive or wandering behavior. Once that bath is completed, the care team need to take immediate steps to decrease that client's anxiety before placing any further demands upon him.

Flexibility during the "Transition Period" is the key to successful admission. This client will probably not undress the first night or two, wandering the halls instead of sleeping. He will then sit when he is tired for short periods in a chair and probably awake more confused, not knowing whether it is day or night. These qualities should not become a point of concern. They are a normal response by the mentally impaired to the changes occurring. Once a degree of familiarity is gained, the care team and family should see a return to a more normal sleeping pattern within a few days.

Likewise, the new client will not be able to handle eating in the dining room the first few meals. Some new clients may require their meals scheduled before or after everyone else, being allowed to eat in the dining room when there is less commotion. For the care team to provide such flexibility, they need a microwave oven on the unit to allow them to reheat the meal when he is hungry. In fact for some new clients, light, frequent meals that can be "eaten on the run" may be the best option.

Finally, the care team needs to withhold unnecessary activities - bath, assessment, large group involvement, etc. - until it is obvious that this client is able to respond to the demands placed upon him. Once there is a decline in anxiety from the initial move to the unit and some degree of familiarity is gained, then gradually introducing the client to the routines of the unit is possible. Staff cannot be so caught up in the routine of getting things done, that they overlook the consequences it creates for the new client. Flexibility, the willingness to try and then back off if the client is obviously stressed by the task, separates units who are effective with this clientele from those who are not.

c) Involving Family

Asking family to assist with certain activities is a significant asset to the care team. Identifying for family when the care team plans to complete a new component of the care routine or postponing a task (i.e. shaving) until family can arrange to visit may decrease for this client much of the anxiety that can be experienced.

The most traumatic time for the new client on any unit is usually the first bath. If possible, caregivers need to schedule the first bath when they are sure they have the time to invest to complete it without being rushed. This allows caregivers the opportunity to provide the needed supports: showing the client the tub room, having her run the water, accompanying the client back to her bedroom to gather her housecoat, and return to the tub room to undress and bathe. It is advantageous to have the initial tub bath completed by the caregiver who has gained the greatest rapport with this client.

If possible, all efforts should be made to have a family member in attendance to assist with that first bath on the unit. If family have cared for this client prior to admission, they have completed that person's bath many times and would now be a stabilizing influence to help the client cope. Even if family have never assisted the client with a tub bath prior to admission, having them on the unit when the bath is completed to assist caregivers in comforting the client is a tremendous asset that will contribute to the caregiver's success.

In each of these examples, staff must assess every aspect of the care routine to determine the best approach or intervention needed. The information gained must then be shared with the care team in the preliminary care plan. Once the new client has settled, the initial care plan can then be updated.

It is always interesting to encounter the responses to the above admission process by some staff and managers. The most frequently heard comment is, "This all sounds nice, but in reality it cannot be done. There is no time to do it."

With any supportive measures discussed throughout this text the choice is a simple one - to do it or not do it. It is the difference between adapting the setting to effectively care for this clientele, or forcing this individual to adapt to an environment in which he cannot function. An environment that is beyond his ability to cope creates for him a detrimental setting in which to live.

Time is not the factor here. No matter what is done or not done, time is a constant. We have demonstrated that not providing the supports identified could result in significant and frequent behavioral outbursts, and resistance by the new client. The consequences of inaction (not setting up the needed supportive measures) can easily be reflected in the wasted caregiver time to control an aggressive client, and the expenditure of energy to settle other clients on the unit who have been influenced by this client's response. Each task that is performed without sensitivity to the person's ability only further elevates that person's anxiety. This now makes the simplest tasks, which could have been completed in a supportive setting, impossible to do.

Investing the time to develop and adhere to a supportive admission procedure will lessen the negative impact of admission and decrease the behavioral responses to a more tolerable level. The time invested in taking the appropriate steps to establish an effective admission process is then saved in the decreased need to deal with intense reactionary behavior by the new admission. In either case, time will be invested. The difference is whether one wants to engage in problem solving or crisis intervention.

The consequences of crisis intervention are always disastrous. Waiting for a crisis to occur only elevates the client's anxiety level and creates a negative behavioral response for an extended period of time. The resultant altercation to that response only upsets other clients on the unit, decreases the ability of staff to perform their care, and jeopardizes the safety of staff and clients concerned. The choice is:

Problem Solving or
Crisis Intervention.

Chapter Eleven

Assessment

Assessment is required to define every aspect of care. However, there are few situations where a client is unable to provide assistance, direct information and/or feedback during an assessment. Of course those with dementia are the exception. The inability of the mentally impaired to analyze, comprehend and/or communicate shifts the assessment to a unilateral investigative process. Assessing the needs of a dementia client requires a comprehensive array or "bag" of assessment tools. Without the appropriate assessment tools, behaviors cannot be managed successfully. The importance of assessment can best be demonstrated by the following:

A detailed and comprehensive assessment process
Defines client specific care practices
Resulting in minimal challenging behaviors
Requiring minimal use of chemical or physical restraints.

No one assessment tool can accomplish what is required to address the complex needs of those with dementia. To be effective and functional, a comprehensive assessment process must incorporate three key components:

1) All involved with the client's care should be directly involved in the assessment process.
2) The assessment tools must be functional.
3) The forms and process used must be adapted to the organization's resources and needs.

It is not necessary for an organization to work from scratch in developing the needed assessment tools, but only to examine the various tools available, and then pull from them what is useful within their setting. There have been a number of assessment procedures identified throughout this text, and in the next few pages even more will be highlighted. Use these in combination with the other assessment tools you are presently using to develop an assessment process that provides the information needed relative to your situation.

Assessment Overview

The objectives of assessment pertaining to the dementia client are in keeping with the principles of Supportive Therapy:

1) Identify what the person is still able to do.
2) Identify what the person is unable to do.
3) Identify the individual's areas of vulnerability.

The key assessment areas include:

- Medical
- Environmental
- Functional (ADL, social, activity, etc.)
- Psychological Profile
- Mental Status
- History
- Medication

Earlier chapters discussed the medical, environmental and mental status assessments. The following chapter will address many of the functional assessment tools. Subsequent chapters are dedicated to care analysis and programming assessment methods.

Medication Assessment/Minimal Restraint

Many progressive organizations (LTC and acute) have adopted a minimal restraint policy. Medication used to manage behavior can be treated no different than any other restraint. Once a minimal restraint policy is incorporated into the care process it must automatically result in dramatic steps to limit the use of medications to manage behavior. To adhere to the principles of a minimal restraint policy, medication assessment needs to focus on four primary areas:

a) New Medication Assessment
b) Three Month Drug Review
c) Trial Period Without
d) 21 Day Maximum Order

a) New Medication Assessment (Acute, LTC, Community, Family)

The challenges in relation to medication usage with the mentally impaired stems from a number of sources:

- At times the treating physician is not the client's original doctor.
- The original symptom that initiated ordering a specific drug may no longer be present.
- Those who influence the ordering of medication may not be experienced with specific clients and their behaviors.
- The functional ability and behavior of many mentally impaired clients can change given certain circumstances and time.
- Specific drugs may build-up to toxic levels gradually over time.
- A long-standing drug may now create problems when combined with another medication.

- The tolerance level of the mentally impaired to medication may be substantially less than the general population of older people.

The sensitivity of the mentally impaired to medication is an ongoing concern. Some medications can cause a gradual build-up, where toxic effects are not demonstrated until the drug has been administered for a considerable period called Cumulative Toxicity.

Drowsiness, altered gait, loss in muscle coordination, changes in ability to perform basic tasks, etc. can all be attributed to administration of a new medication, or alteration in dosage or dispensing frequency of existing medication. Unfortunately these changes can be disregarded, mistakenly attributing them to the progressive nature of the disease, rather than a direct side effect of the medication used.

It is direct line caregivers who can best monitor a client's functioning ability from one day to the next. Line staff must understand their role in monitoring drug use with this clientele. Even though their knowledge of specific drugs may be limited, their assessment is critical. All members of the care team must be encouraged to vocalize suspected changes in a client's functioning and allowed to question whether a drug is helping or hindering a client's abilities. An ideal New Medication Policy establishes the following assessment procedure:

- Direct caregivers are to monitor and record any changes in the client's ability and/or functioning for one month after dosage or frequency of an existing medication is initiated or a new medication is ordered.
- All new medication orders or changes to existing medication made within the past month are to be reviewed at the care conference to determine the impact on the client.

These steps are essential to monitor gradual and less obvious side effects to medication. The next step is to monitor and eliminate existing medication utilizing the Three Month Review and the Trial Period Without.

b) Three Month Drug Review (Acute, LTC)

The best philosophy concerning drug usage is *'When in doubt, do without. When in use, use the minimum.'* Given the sensitivity of this clientele to medication, regular monitoring by the physician and care team is essential. Considering that very little is known about the effects of one drug on any one client, a combination of six, eight or ten in a twenty-four hour period becomes a major concern.

A commonly used drug assessment process is the Three Month Drug Review. In order to ensure that this review has some clout and drugs are not simply rewritten every three months without being scrutinized, a policy must be established that dictates:

An automatic stop order on all drugs every three months.

Any drug can be re-ordered, but it must be treated as a new order. This requires the physician to write the order on the Doctor's Order Sheet and also write the reason the drug is to be continued in the Doctor's Progress Notes. This can be simplified. Drugs related specifically to a client's diagnosis are easily dealt with. If the client is on Aldomet for hypertension and Diabeta for diabetes, then he simply writes in the doctor's progress notes:

Aldomet (see medical)
Diabeta (see medical)

The drugs being challenged by this process are the non-life threatening medications such as the hypnotics and sedatives. These are drugs that have been ordered primarily to deal with behavioral issues.

When reviewing any medication, one simple question needs to be asked of the physician before she re-writes the order:

"Doctor, what would happen if we took that drug and decreased the dosage, or stopped the drug all together?"

If she answers, "You can't do that or this will happen . . .", she has just given the rationale for why that drug must be continued. If she answers, "I don't know!", then she has just initiated the next assessment tool required - the Trial Period Without.

c) The Trial Period Without (Acute, LTC, Community)

If a mentally impaired client demonstrates considerable aggressive behavior and frequently attempts to leave the building on admission, does it mean that after six months of living on the unit he will still be aggressive and attempt to leave the building?

(Note: It is assumed in discussing this case that all necessary measures have been taken to determine that the aggressive and elopement behavior demonstrated cannot be minimized by any other supportive measure other than medication.)

There are three possible answers.

1) He can be <u>worse</u>. His aggressive outbursts and attempts to leave the building have increased since admission. In that case no medication has been found to be effective, and the care team as tested different types of drugs, dosages, etc. along with a variety of other supportive measures with no success. There is no use considering that person for the Trial Period Without.

2) This client's aggression seems to have <u>leveled,</u> where the medication being dispensed and the supportive measures being used are just holding the behavior under control. He is still

having periodic outbursts, but it is considered by all to be too early to take this client off his medication.

3) However, the possibility is just as high that this client would no longer be aggressive or attempt to leave the building, even if he were off the medication.

The aggressive and elopement behavior may no longer be present for two reasons. The first is that the disease may have progressed to the point where he no longer has the ability to be aggressive. The second is that he may have gained sufficient familiarity with the staff, routines and unit over the past six months to decrease his anxiety level and eliminate the aggressive response. In either case, why is he still on the original medication ordered to control that behavior?

A very effective assessment mechanism to determine if specific non-life threatening medications - sedatives, hypnotics, anti-anxiety agents, etc. are still needed is the Trial Period Without. If over the last two months there has not been a recurrence of the original symptoms that initiated the medication, or the physician does not know the effect if a dosage is lowered or the drug is discontinued, then the client is tried without that drug or with a lower dose for a period of four to eight weeks (the appropriate length will depend on the half life of the specific medication).

It is advisable that a back-up PRN (to be given as needed) sedation be ordered during this time if necessary. If there is no behavioral change during the trial period, then the medication is discontinued or the dosage is decreased further. Once there is some indication of a behavioral change (increased restlessness, greater difficulty to complete care tasks, etc.), then the drug can be elevated slightly, indicating that the most therapeutic dose for this client has been reached.

It is important when implementing such a program that one medication be attempted at a time. If two or more drugs are experimented with and specific behaviors recur, it will be impossible to determine which drug is needed and which is not.

It is crucial that all members of the care team be involved in the client's behavioral and functional assessment during the trial period. Having a client in a "full blown" agitated state eight days after the drug has been decreased or removed, requires considerable energies and resources to calm him and negatively impacts the rest of the unit. Direct line staff (care aides, housekeepers, activity staff, etc.) must report any changes observed - increased restlessness, difficult to toilet, harder to perform personal care, unable to sit for any length of time, etc., when they occur.

The information provided by direct line staff is important for two reasons. First, identifying any subtle changes in behavior may provide the necessary warning of a potential increase in agitation that may require the medication to be re-instated. Secondly, it helps to determine if there is any improvement in the client's functioning or behavior now that the medication has been decreased or stopped.

Summary of Trial Period Without

1) The behavior that initiated ordering the medication has not been seen within the past two months, or the physician does not have a sound rationale for re-ordering it.

2) The drug is stopped or dosage decreased for a period of four to eight weeks (depending on the half life of the specific medication).

3) A back-up PRN (as needed) sedative is ordered in case the behavior returns during the trial period and threatens to become uncontrollable.

4) All members of the care team are required to report and record behavioral and/or functional changes noted during this time, whether better or worse.

5) If the originating behavior does not recur during the trial
period, the back-up PRN sedative is discontinued, the original
drug is stopped, or in the case where the dosage was lowered,
it is lowered further.

21 Day Maximum Order (Acute, LTC)

To adhere to a minimal restraint philosophy, psychotropic
medication, drugs used to manage behaviors, must be treated as any
other restraint. Implementation must be restricted, with continuous
investigation to find alternate supportive measures. Implementation of
a 21 Day Maximum Order (the time restriction can vary depending on
the severity of the case in question) is necessary to achieve the
desired results.

A 21 Day Maximum Order requires the care team to investigate
alternative solutions other than psychotropic medication. If alternative
action is taken and the behavior is managed then the drug is decreased
or discontinued. If the behavior persists, the drug is renewed for
another 21 days during which time the care team is required to
summon the assistance of other specialists or disciplines (physician,
psychiatrist or psycho-geriatrician, behavioral specialist, etc.).

At no time is the care team allowed to become complacent
regarding medication used for behavior. This approach ensures that
the care team continually investigates alternate supportive measures
other than medication to manage behaviors. When the expectation is
minimal restraint without exception, no psychotropic medication can
be ordered without ongoing assessment. This is not unlike the steps
taken when a physical restraint is ordered.

The 24 Hour Profile (Acute, LTC, Community, Family)

This tool has had the most dramatic impact in managing
challenging behaviors. The intention of the 24 Hour Profile is to
create consistency in care by replicating caregiver success. The tool's

primary objective is to uncover "caregiver secrets." The concept of Caregiver Secrets is well defined in the book Preventing Alzheimer's Aggression. A secret is information known by a caregiver that allows a degree of success that is not known by others. This information is not intentionally held. It is often believed that other caregivers know and therefore not communicated. Two simple facts make the 24 Hour Profile an essential tool for any care team:

- No one caregiver can know any one client totally (what she is capable of doing, how she behaves, etc.) twenty-four hours per day, seven days a week.
- No one caregiver can know what the rest of the team does that is successful with all clients on the unit each shift.

The 24 Hour Profile is key to ensuring that information is collected and communicated to all involved with a specific client. The information generated from the 24 Hour Profile creates the intervention column of the client care plan and becomes the basis for the Care Plan Summary (see chapter on Care Analysis). This tool is effective for all disciplines, it is:

- ideal for LTC or acute care, to be completed on existing clients or on any new admission
- effective for community support to be completed by all caregivers involved with the client
- a must for family caregivers (the headings day shift need to be changed to day time and evening/night shift to evening/night time) when admitting the family member to LTC, Acute Care, a Dementia Day Program or utilizing community support

The following is an overview of the actual document, how to use the tool and examples of its effectiveness.

The 24 Hour Profile

This is a *solutions oriented* assessment tool. DO NOT expand on the care issues (problems or concerns) encountered. Provide only successful strategies employed or information known about the client, regarding each of the identified care issues.

The intention of the following assessment is to provide a profile of a specific client's functioning level over a 24 hour period. The goal of this information is to:

1) Identify changes in functioning noticed between shifts (days, afternoons and nights).
2) Identify the client's strengths and limitations.
3) Identify successful techniques or approaches employed by certain caregivers in each area.

(Note: Only the questionnaire section of the 24 Hour Profile is presented in these pages. The complete questionnaire is located in the appendix at the back of the book. What is missing is the space to check off "Yes" or "No" for each statement and the supportive data section that is completed by day, afternoon and night shift.)

Instructions

Step One
This questionnaire is to be initiated by a caregiver who best knows the client to be assessed. That caregiver is required to complete the Supportive Data section for the shift that she has most contact with this client (day, evening or night shift). Be as specific as possible, recording any supportive data you believe appropriate to describe this individual's functioning in each area. Remember the goal is to replicate what you are doing, provide detailed description. In the space under Supportive Data include the following:

- pattern of behavior (time of day, equipment to be set in a specific
   manner, specific items used, etc.).
- when have you seen changes (will or will not function)?
- what do you say or do to the client to assist the person to function?
- effective means to encourage the person to function?
- how can you tell if the individual is being pressured and it is best not to attempt the task at this time?

Step Two
The completed form is then reviewed by each shift (day, evening and night), adding to the information provided.

Step Three
Once completed, a list of care issues are extracted, and the guidelines outlined in the supportive data section providing the basis for the care plan.

Assessment
Client Being Assessed: _____
Initial Assessment Completed by: _____
Date of Initial Assessment: _____
Date Reviewed by Day Shift: _____
Date Reviewed by Evening Shift: _____
Date Reviewed by Night Shift: _____

Important: Identify solutions only, be detailed and specific. The goal is to replicate what you do!

Activities of Daily Living
   1) Mealtime
- needs assistance?
- easily distracted?
   (if yes, how is this dealt with?)

- can only handle a few items at a time?
      (if yes, which & in what order?)
- any special arrangement or items?

2) Hygiene
a) Bathing
- cooperative in tub?
      (if no, explain.)
- needs assistance?
- any special arrangements or items?

b) Teeth/Hair
- needs assistance?
- requires articles to be handed to him/her?
- only requires articles be displayed?
- cooperative during procedure?
      (if no, explain?)
- any special arrangements or items?

c) Dressing
- requires assistance dressing or undressing?
- requires articles to be displayed?
- requires articles to be handed to him/her?
- problems with specific articles of clothing?
- can pick own clothing from closet?
- any special arrangements or items?

d) Toileting
- specific times? (which?)
- needs to be checked? (when?)
- how does he/she communicate the need to go to
    the washroom (does he tell you or by what actions)?
- any special arrangements or items?

3) Ambulation
- gait unsteady (describe gait)

- needs to be checked, will exhaust self?
      (what time of day and what is done if unsteady?)
- wanders? (identify time and specific area)
- how do you deal with the wandering?

Comprehension

- understands instructions? (if no, explain)
- responds to his/her name? (first, last or nickname)
- can identify staff or family members?
      (who and how often?)
- can identify all objects? (if no, what and when?)
- finds way around unit?
      (room, washroom, dining room, lounge)
- what must you do to help this person understand
   what you are saying or what you want done?

Behavior

In each area where (yes) is checked describe what the client does
and how you deal with it:
- restlessness
- repetitive behavior destructive
- needs assistance?
- disturbing behavior (who?)
- hoarding (what, from where?)
- verbally/physically threatening others

Social Skills

- can relate to others?
     (will talk to who, when and about what?)
- helps others? (who & when?)
- relates well to new people? (if no, explain what happens)
- participates in group activities? (what and when?)

Activities

>   - performs specific chores on the unit? (what and when?)
>   - involved in specific games, hobbies?
>   (what, when and for how long?)
>   - reads or looks through books/magazines?
>   - enjoys music, TV (what and when?)

****

Using The 24 Hour Profile

As outlined in Step One, the form is initiated by the caregiver who experiences less of a problem or no problem with this individual (or by the family member if the person is in the community or just being admitted). This individual usually knows many of the "secrets" pertaining to the client being assessed and is often the best to initiate the assessment.

It is important when using the 24 Hour Profile to emphasize that this is a working document. Caregivers with limited formal education or writing ability may be reluctant to contribute. It is not necessary to be able to write effectively or spell properly, the goal is to gain the information needed to develop a client centered care plan and care plan summary. Likewise, it is important that information be specific and detailed. Using words such as usual, normal, etc. provide little direction. Others reading the information must be able to replicate what is outlined.

The form does not need to be completed within 24 hours but represents 24 hours. Once the initial caregiver completes the form it is then passed to other caregivers for their input. In LTC and acute care, the completed form is given to the care team on the day shift, then that completed form is passed to evening shift for their input and that form then passed to night shift. All staff of all departments who have contact with the client in question must have input. Information from the completed form is then extrapolated to develop the intervention column of the care plan and the care plan summary.

Examples of Information Gained

Once completed, the 24 Hour Profile provides considerable insight into this client's performance, needs and abilities. An example that demonstrates the benefits of this tool involved a client named Ann.

Ann's cognitive ability was very limited and her attention span extremely short. All caregivers found it difficult to toilet this lady. When staff sat her on the toilet she would immediately stand up. The sitting-standing was constant until she would urinate on the floor. All caregivers agreed with the problem, but no solution was known until the afternoon conference reviewed her 24 Hour Profile.

A part-time caregiver stated that she had no difficulty toileting this lady. She found a song that Ann liked to sing. She would begin singing the song with Ann while she was standing in front of the toilet. She would then ease her to the toilet still singing. While Ann sat on the toilet, the caregiver stood in front of her with her knees against Ann's knees and her face close to Ann's singing the song with her. This stalled Ann long enough to have her urinate in the toilet. A simple solution to a complex problem.

The information generated by the 24 Hour Profile is quite revealing and extremely valuable. However, the care team must become practiced at using this tool so that the information is client centered, specific and detailed enough that it is replicable.

The Interview(Acute, LTC, Community)

Unfortunately, many direct line caregivers do not often use the interview as a formal assessment process with a level two mentally impaired client. Considerable information can be gained from interviewing an individual at this level of functioning. To conduct a successful interview, the interviewer must establish a degree of rapport with the client.

Before any client can be interviewed, all information about that client must be obtained from the caregivers involved (staff and/or family). Asking caregivers the following questions is essential:

Where is the best place to meet this person?
When is this person's best times of the day?
When is this person's worst times of the day?
What topics of discussion does the client not tolerate?
What topics of discussion does the client enjoy?
How do you know when the client is becoming distressed?
What can be done or said to decrease the client's distress?
How does the client respond to touch?
Is it important that someone new be introduced by a familiar staff
    member?
Would this client respond better to an interview if a familiar staff
    member was present?
How long can this person sit with others?
How long can this person be attentive to a conversation?
How would you know it was too long?

Not knowing what cues to read, what can or cannot be tolerated, etc.,
will negatively effect the results of the interview.

The interview can determine:

- attention span
- emotional state
- language pattern
- thought process

Attention span

The interview must be conducted in a quiet location, free from
unnecessary noise and stimuli. The more familiar the environment to
the client, the better (usually her room with the door closed). This
ensures the client is not distracted by other noise and movement. If
the client is unable to concentrate on what is being said, or to sit
longer than a few moments without getting restless, then that is a
significant indication of the client's attention span. If she is unable to
concentrate on this very direct and intense stimuli, then she will have

considerable difficulty lasting in any activity that is longer than a few moments.

Defining the client's attention span is important information for the care team. When identified, caregivers can then be directed on the strategies to employ to compensate for this person's poor attention span (defining attention is valuable when completing a Shadow Assessment and ADL Map – see following section).

Emotional state

It is important for the interviewer to uncover the emotional overtones of the client's conversation. The emotional state of a mentally impaired client can be expressed in many indirect ways. The client talking about this place as a prison, or the one who is suspicious during the interview provides considerable insight into the person's needs. If the individual's anxiety level is high, the emotions expressed will be ones of fear. In this case, the care team must be directed on ways to establish rapport and security in order to lessen the feelings encountered.

Language pattern

The interviewer must be attentive, listening to the pattern of words during the conversation will give an indication of any language deficiencies. For example, using the word "brother" instead of "husband" demonstrates such a loss. It may indicate that the person has forgotten her husband's name or her relationship to him, and she has replaced "husband" with the next nearest word - "brother." This process is called *word replacement*. Once this is uncovered, then staff need to be directed to identify any patterns of other words that may be consistently used out of context (i.e. "rag" for face cloth, or "scoop" for "spoon"). This information must be placed on the care plan and communicated to all staff in contact with this client.

Thought process

Some mentally impaired clients can experience disjointed thoughts, where each phrase expressed has no apparent relationship to the other - "The moon is in the sky. I saw the chickens. Where's my daughter?"

Although it may appear that the client is unable to respond to questions or carry on any type of conversation, this may not be the case. When this is encountered, it is important for the interviewer to determine:

- if this client is capable of responding appropriately to yes/no questions.
- if, in all of the rambling the client does stop, responds appropriately to the question asked, and then continues rambling.
- if a recurrent theme or thought process is intermixed within the rambling. Weed through the excess, and you may find the person has some logic to the thoughts expressed.

In each of these cases, caregivers must be given direction on how to communicate to the client rather than assume that she cannot respond.

Reminiscing

It is important during an interview not only to listen for the right answers to the questions being asked, but also to what the client is talking about. Much of her conversation may be out of context to what is being discussed, but if you listen to what she is saying, it may be logical - she talks of her daughter when she was fourteen and is very accurate in her description of that past event. This lady becomes an excellent candidate for reminiscing. The care team can be instructed to carry on a conversation about her past and be fairly confident that the information she is sharing is accurate. Staff may also be successful in performing a process called *progressive orientation* - filling in the gaps, by talking to her about the time she believes it is, then moving her forward to the present - "Your daughter went to high school, didn't she? Then college . . . she got married . . . she has children."

Set precedent

What is more significant about having the interview as part of the assessment process is the expectation it sets for the care team:

Regardless of the mental functioning level of a client,
it is expected that all caregivers will communicate
with every mentally impaired client.

This fosters an understanding that a mentally impaired client still needs to be heard, and considerable information can be gained from what the client says.

History (Acute, LTC, Community, Family)

Family are the key to successfully caring for the mentally impaired elderly. In fact, family members who have cared for their parent prior to admission are even more valuable. They may have already found what works and what causes problems concerning mother's care. Not to tap that information immediately means that the care team will go through the same trial and error process, needlessly distressing the client and being ineffective in their care.

Family can often help fill in the "blanks" by not only giving us a clear picture of how they have cared for mother since she became impaired, but also of who mother was before the onset of the disease. A family questionnaire (outlined in the previous chapter) is essential.

The more we can understand who that client was before the onset of the disease and what has occurred prior to admission, the better equipped we will be in establishing an environment specific to the needs of that person. Once the information is obtained, it is shared with the team and incorporated into the care plan.

Shadow Assessment (Acute, LTC, Community)

Generally caregivers will postpone care when a client is obviously uncooperative or unwilling to perform, called Global Flexibility. Although successful with most clients, it may not be adequate enough for those with challenging behaviors. The more challenging client requires a more defined approach called Focused Flexibility.

To develop Focused Flexibility requires the care team to determine exactly the timing and order tasks should be completed. This is defined by conducting a Shadow Assessment and creating an ADL Map. The following example will demonstrate these tools.

In one case example, staff identified that a male client became aggressive while removing his pants and changing his incontinent briefs. A Shadow Assessment was conducted to determine the contributing factors to his behavioral response and the required supportive measures. A Shadows Assessment involves shadowing or observing a caregiver in action and creating an ADL Map. An ADL Map defines the following:

- what the client is experiencing.
- the potential rational for the task and the impact on the client.
- possible alternative actions that can be taken.

The following are the results of the Shadow Assessment completed on the client in question:

ADL Map

Action	Rational or Impact	Alternate Approach
The client was wandering down the hall.	His ritualistic behavior, utilizes wandering to alleviate anxiety.	
Two staff approached him from behind.	Staff were concerned about his aggressive history. Two approach in case he may strike. Client becomes startled and overwhelmed by the contact.	One should approach and the other out of view in case needed. Frontal approach at angle from dominate side instead of from behind.

Action	Rational or Impact	Alternate Approach
He was stopped.	Stopping without warning is a restraining action that appeared to increase his anxiety.	Walk with him allowing his thought process to catch up with caregiver's actions stopping him gradually if needed.
Both staff spoke to him.	Client bombarded and confused, looking from one staff member to the other in attempt to understand.	One caregiver approaching him eliminates the problem.
He was turned around to take him down the hall.	Abrupt directional change confused the client resulting in his pulling back and resisting staff.	Walk with a more gradual change in direction. Diverting him with appropriate topic of conversation.
Entered his room.	All rooms are similar to the next, client stalled at the door to see if it was his room, staff not aware of his stall and moved him before he could orientate himself.	Stall at door to give him time to see familiar objects, point out objects if needed.
One staff member sat him on the bedside.		
Other staff member entered his bathroom.	Could not see second staff member once she walked away, could only hear noises but not understand where they were coming from and by whom.	Having second staff member standing in hallway by the door would eliminate this stimuli and confusion.
Removed his shirt and undershirt.	Based on staff interviews, staff who knew him stated that he did not like being cold, not known by others.	Require 24 Hour Profile and Care Plan Summary to identify remove shirt and undershirt, wash quickly and re-dress.

Action	Rational or Impact	Alternate Approach
Staff member placed the bedside table in front of him.	Became confused, did not know what it was, obviously felt blocked in or restrained.	Place bedside table to the side of him, still in view and accessible but not confining him.
Other staff member brought a basin of water from the bathroom and placed it in front of him.	Could not relate to the bedside table and basin of water.	Needed to be placed in front of a sink or at least accompany staff into the bathroom to fill the basin of water.
Staff member in front of him handed him a face cloth to wash his face and hands.	Could not relate to what was being asked.	Same as above
Other staff member stood behind him.	Did not know she was there increasing his confusion.	Second staff member should be outside the door and ready to assist if needed.
Given towel to dry his face.		
General conversation with him.	Irrelevant conversation, could not relate to the topic, respond or hold his attention.	Topic must be specific to client's interest and history to divert and decrease anxiety.
Periodic conversation staff to staff.	He would answer when staff spoke to the co-worker behind him, became very confused.	Conversation should be directed to client only.
Other staff stood behind to wash his back.	Reality shock, no warning of her presence. Bombarding, too much stimuli from too many sources.	One caregiver to provide care only, with other ready to assist if needed.

Action	Rational or Impact	Alternate Approach
Staff member in front of him placed shaving lather on his face, she was wearing latex gloves.	Latex gloves confused him, he could not recognize her hands.	The need to use latex gloves must be restricted to clients with a high risk for AIDS. Not necessary with this client.
Staff shaved him while standing in front of him.	He could not see her hands and had no warning when she was placing the razor to his face.	Sit down at right angles to him allows him to see her hand come up to his face.
Dried his face with a towel.		
Washed under his arms.		
Applied deodorant.	No assessment whether this individual used role on, spray or any deodorant at all.	Should be assessment question when completing history. Apparently, man did not use deodorant and other staff stated not required, minimal body odor.
Put on his undershirt and shirt.	Too long before he was covered.	See above.
Stood him up.		
Removed his pants.	No conversation other than telling him what was being done.	Need to discuss topic relevant to this client to distract him from the task being completed.
Removed his incontinent briefs.	The task that created the most difficulty.	

Action	Rational or Impact	Alternate Approach
If he is not aggressive, staff would instruct him to do his own peri-care.	Commonly aggressive.	
If he is aggressive, then the other staff would assist.	Usually resulting in significant aggressive behavior, second staff member attempting to restrain his hands while the other struggled with his pants and incontinent briefs. All other tasks from this point on were difficult to complete. Staff moved quickly in order to get everything done, only contributing to his agitation.	
Put on his pants.		
Did his belt, zipper, combed his hair.		
Put on his shoes, glasses and hat.	Client now wandered the hall in an aggressive state, psychotropic PRN medication often administered as a result.	

The a result of the Shadow Assessment generated the following questions:

Why would all tasks – washing, undressing, dressing, shaving, changing his incontinent pads, etc. be done together as though they were one task?

If the most difficult task is removing his pants and changing his incontinent briefs, why would that be intertwined with all other tasks?

The number of stressors encountered before the most demanding task (changing his incontinent briefs) increased the risk of an aggressive response.

Clients demonstrating challenging behaviors require the care team to identify the care task(s) that will trigger the most intense behavioral response, then separate that task from any other demands. This is called Focused Flexibility. Once determined, the order of those tasks and the way they are approached are outlined in the intervention column of the care plan and summarized on the Care Plan Summary. In this way the sequence, time frame, approach, etc. is specific to the client's abilities and vulnerabilities. Once defined and consistently integrated into the care routine, the frequency and duration of challenging behaviors will be decreased.

Assessing Behavior Risk (Acute, LTC)

If a client had serious cardiac problems that require close observation, would there not be discussion during the report at each shift change on what should be done or was needed over the next eight hours to address that issue? A client demonstrating challenging behaviors has the same requirement. It is surprising how often a behavioral issue experienced by the previous shift is raised during report at shift change, yet there is no further discussion of how that behavior is to be addressed during the next shift. When caring for those with challenging behaviors, problem solving must be a continuous team process.

Shift report is the opportunity for the care team to problem solve on what preventative measures are needed over the next eight hours. At the beginning of each shift, the care team:

- must identify those clients demonstrating high risk challenging behaviors (aggression, aggressive wanderer, ingestion of foreign substances, choking, high elopement risk, etc.).
- review care strategies required for these clients.
- discuss the emotional state of these clients as reported from the last shift.
- identify potential risk factors that may exist for the upcoming shift.
- determine strategies or interventions required to eliminate or decrease those risks.

Likewise, at the end of each shift, the shift leader (RN or RPN) must meet with the care team to identify any new information or strategies uncovered (to be added to the care plan and care plan summary) or potential risk factors for the next shift. This provides needed information for the next shift to repeat the process. In this way it is not left up to one caregiver (the one assigned this client) the sole responsibility to determine what is needed or to wait until the behavior demonstrates itself before it is addressed. Problem solving that results in preventive care creates the desired outcome.

Behavioral Incident Assessment (Acute, LTC, Community, Family)

One of the basic concepts identified in earlier chapters established the following:

The dementia client always communicates, not verbally but by behavior. Understand the behavioral cues as they apply to the specific client will provide the needed direction on how to support the client and manage the behavior.

Knowing that the dementia client communicates by behavior, it is essential to re-create or assess each behavioral episode. Examining what occurred will often identify what triggered the behavior and the supportive measures required to resolve it. However, if the assessment is open-ended, based on the caregiver's ability, the resultant information may be of little value. The Behavioral Incident Assessment is a comprehensive tool that provides direction on how to analyze a behavioral episode. This form is completed after an intense behavioral response by those witnessing the episode.

Behavioral Incident Assessment (Acute, LTC, Community, Family)

Date: _____
Time Behavior Witnessed: _____
Client's Name: _____
Behavior Observed: _____
Completed By: _____
Caregiver(s) Witnessing _____
    the Episode:

Complete the following assessment on the most recent incident.

- Describe in detail the actions of the client during the incident in question (what the client did or said).

- Did the client direct the behavior towards anyone or anything specifically: Yes No

    If Yes, identify the person(s) or thing(s)?

- Identify what was going on around or to the person at that time.

- Who was in contact with or around the client when the behavior occurred?

- Where was the client and what was the client doing prior to the incident?

- How long did the behavioral response last?

- What was the client like after the incident in question?

- What did the client do after the incident in question and where did the client go?

- Identify anything different about the environment, the individual's routine, medication used, etc. at the time or on the day of the incident.

- Identify how the situation could have been handled differently.

The information generated by the Behavioral Incident Assessment will provide significant direction on the supportive measures required. It is important that these forms not be used independently, but collectively. Whenever BIA forms are completed, whether they are for the same behavioral response or different behaviors, they should always be compared. When the information in one form is compared to another, patterns will emerge providing significant direction on what may be specific triggers for the client in question and what is required.

Assessment is an ongoing process. The emphasis begins on first contact and continues for as long as we are caring for the client. Given that our role is to advocate for the client, the assessment process and the information generated must have defined internal and external policies and procedures, a Behavior Care Practices Manual. Internal policies and procedures identify when each tool is to be used and how the information generated is analyzed and communicated (i.e. care conference, care plan and care plan summary).

However, if the tools and information generated is essential for your organization to perform care, then it is essential for all in contact with the client. The Behavior Care Practices Manual containing forms, guidelines on how they are analyzed and communicated must accompany all transfers. Not only is the information valuable to provide the direction on what to do with this client, it also provides direction on what is needed for all with dementia. In fact, some make it a requirement. No admission or transfer is allowed without this information being provided. Imagine the impact of all three specialty areas (LTC, acute care and community) utilized similar practices. Each would build on the other to generate the information required and the care strategies to support the client - a highly effective care system that addresses the uniqueness of those with dementia.

Chapter Twelve

Behavior Analysis

There is no question that those with dementia are highly complex. Yet some caregivers still have the tendency to limit their expectations of a client's behavior to simple answers to describe a very complex problem.

There is nothing more disheartening than to have individuals over-simplify the behaviors of the mentally impaired. We have spent considerable time describing the complexities of this clientele, the gray areas that are not clearly or easily visible. These are the issues that must be uncovered in order to gain the necessary direction for our care.

No matter what client behavior is discussed, there is <u>always</u> an underlying cause. Until that cause is defined, there is no effective supportive measure that can be employed to successfully manage the behavior other than a form of physical or chemical restraint. The earlier analysis of wandering and sexual expressive behaviors were not presented to simply define different causes for each of these behaviors. The potential causes become the foundation from which to conduct a highly specific and very basic behavioral management technique called Behavior Analysis.

Behavior Analysis involves three components:

- An analytical process to determine the underlying cause of a behavior (Care Analysis).

- An ability to communicate client specific supportive measures to all in contact with the client to ensure consistency (Care Plan Summary).

- An ongoing assessment and analysis of the results of the supportive measures taken (Success Oriented Charting).

As each of the tools of Behavior Analysis are outlined (Care Analysis, Care Plan Summary, Success Oriented Charting), the related assessment tools (see section on Assessment) that contribute to the analysis process are also identified.

Care Analysis (LTC, acute, community)
Links: Admission Assessment, Behavioral Incident Assessment,   Interview,
Shadow Assessment, Patterning

Care Analysis is a basic behavioral analysis technique used to define the causative factors creating a specific behavior. Utilized during the care conference, it allows the care team to brainstorm what may be causing a client's behavior or change in functioning. The steps in Care Analysis are as follows:

- A formal mechanism utilized during the care conference.
- At the care conference, a flip chart is placed in front of the group and a caregiver is asked to become the recorder.
- The recorder writes on the flip chart a concern or behavior (called a care issue) regarding the client being discussed (i.e. wandering, aggression, hoarding, etc.).
- Members of the care conference are required to identify all possible causes that may create the behavior. The recorder writes each cause on the flip chart sheet.
- Once all causes are recorded, the care team is to identify which cause they believe applies to the client in question.
- Once defined, the potential cause is then written as the Care Diagnosis on the client care plan.

Each of the behaviors defined earlier (wandering and sexual behavior) is best analyzed utilizing this method. For example, if a client is wandering, then wandering is placed at the top of the flip chart. All possible reasons for that behavior are listed. The flip chart sheet would appear as follows:

<u>Wandering</u>
Mimicking
Looking for something familiar
Investigative Wandering
Fear/Anxiety/Stress
Bored
Poor Attention Span
Increased Energy
Medication/Washroom Location
Lifestyle
External Cueing
Physical Discomfort

Invariably the list would be more detailed than the general categories identified above. Once the list is complete, the care team identifies the cause that may apply to the client being discussed. For example, if the primary caregivers felt that the person was bored, then the care plan would identify:

Wandering possibly related to boredom.

The discussion would then center on developing a plan of action to address the issue identified.

Care Analysis is an essential behavioral care investigative process. Determining the accuracy of the defined cause or the effectiveness of the supportive measures implemented is based on the response of the client. If there is no change in the frequency, intensity and/or duration of the behavior, then the cause identified may not be accurate or the supportive measures not sufficient. If there is a noted change in the frequency, intensity and/or duration of the behavior then the direction taken is appropriate.

This analysis process involves a degree of trial and error until the right cause or causes are defined. More than one cause may be a contributing factor, requiring care analysis to be completed on more than one occasion until the client's response validates the supportive measures taken.

Care Analysis Reference
Defining each cause for each behavior during every care conference is not necessary. Creating a Care Analysis Reference section with a Behavioral Care Practices Binder expedites the process. Each behavior is listed alphabetically within the reference section or the practices binder. Once a behavior is analyzed and the causative factors are identified on the flip chart they are recorded in the reference section of the binder under that behavior. When that behavior is to be analyzed again, then the causes listed within the binder are transferred to the flip chart where the care team is asked for additional causes beyond the defined list. Additions are added to the reference binder.

Creating a Care Analysis Reference section within a Behavior Care Practices Binder has a number of benefits:

- continually expands the list of causes as knowledge and expertise increases.
- provides a comprehensive analysis.
- saves time.
- allows those not present at the care conference to add their comments to the analysis process about a specific client.
- expands the insights and understanding of those attending the conference.
- re-familiarizes the causes to those who are not frequently involved with the care conference and care analysis process.

- provides an excellent reference document used during staff orientation and training to understand the behaviors of the mentally impaired elderly.

It is important that the care team develop their own Care Analysis Reference materials. This allows the content of the binder to match the knowledge level of the care team, make the information site specific and creates ownership for what was generated.

Care Plan Summary (LTC, acute, community, family)
Links: 24 Hour Profile, Programming Map, Assessing Behavior Risk,
Behavioral Incident Assessment, Interview, Shadow Assessment

Consistency, flexibility and creativity are the primary care components of behavior management. To achieve consistency, it is essential that all who are in contact with the client are knowledgeable of the specific supportive measures required.

The following case provides an excellent example of how to measure the level of consistency in any care setting. Frank was a dementia client in a long term care setting who would continually call out during meal time and repeatedly attempt to leave the table before he completed his meal. Five caregivers were assembled who said they knew Frank well: a registered nurse, personal care worker, housekeeper, recreation and dietary. One of the five was brought into a conference room while the others were asked to wait in the hall. The caregiver in the conference room was asked:

How do you approach Frank?
How do you get him to the dining room?
How do you get him to sit down?
How do you get him to eat his meal?
What do you do when he becomes upset or disruptive?

The response by this caregiver to the first question was, "You always make your first contact with him from a distance, call his name to get his attention and then come close to him. He hates people coming close to him too quickly."

A second caregiver was brought into the conference room and asked the same questions. Her response to the first question was, "You always approach him from the side, touch him, smile and then state his name." Each of the five caregivers were asked the same set of questions. The majority of their answers were significantly different. It is not surprising that the care team had difficulty with this client and encountered dramatic swings in the effectiveness of the supportive measures implemented.

The challenge for this setting, which is common in many, is word-of-mouth communication. Word-of-mouth communication is a frequent contributing factor to the lack of success in managing most challenging behaviors. It creates two primary obstacles:

1) Information not received
Those who struggle due to word-of-mouth communication are part time, casual, and float nursing staff, as well as others who have less frequent contact with the client (recreation, housekeeping, management, dietary, and other support services). When sporadic or periodic contact with a client is made, it is impossible to remember or know the specific idiosyncrasies for each client. Word-of-mouth communication creates a simple dynamic: the further away a caregiver is from the initiation of the information, the less she will know what is required.

Given the shift-to-shift turnover of caregivers, it is impossible to repeat to everyone on each shift the details of care for every client they are assigned or in contact. It is common for caregivers to work from an intuitive level, doing what is believed to be right. Only to hear, "That is not how we do that with her!" Being told what was required after it is evident that the client is distressed or the challenging behavior is initiated is a little late.

2) Information distorted
We have identified the varying levels of caregiver skills. Some are highly intuitive, able to grasp the concepts of care easily, others are

less intuitive, struggling to uncover or even understand the same information. When word-of-mouth is the primary method of communication, information that is passed on is often subjectively interpreted by each caregiver. To demonstrate, ask five caregivers what supportive means. You will invariably receive five different answers.

Word-of-mouth communication creates subjective care. When information is not made available or the information provided is not accurate then it is impossible to replicate care performance for each client. The result is obvious:

Poor communication creates lack of consistency $\Rightarrow$ Lack of consistency decreases the effectiveness of supportive measures $\Rightarrow$ Ineffective supportive measures initiates challenging behavior.

An effective communication tool in behavior analysis is the Care Plan Summary. This document provides a quick reference on current care information for a specific client. The Care Plan Summary addresses four information areas:

- Base line data
- Stressor profile
- Daily log
- Need to Know

Base Line Data
The first section of the Care Plan Summary identifies specific care requirements in the areas of ADL (activities of daily living). It is not intended to merely list that the client can or cannot perform in these areas. Instead, this section replicates the specific direction on how to assist the client as outlined by the 24 Hour Profile. In the example where the client had difficulty during toileting, the care plan summary would indicate (a sample Care Plan Summary form is located within the addendum):

Base Line Data*: Identify specific care requirements in each of these areas, expand on pertinent data or approaches in the Need to Know section.*

Toileting: Sing "You are my Sunshine",   Bathing   _____
    lower to toilet, place knees against   Teeth/Dentures _____
    knees and face close to client's face,   Glasses   _____
    keep singing until client is done.   Other   _____

Dressing _____
Transfer _____
Mobility _____
Mealtime _____

If more space is required, further information can be added to the Need to Know Section at the bottom of the form. If there is still not enough space for all of the details (which may be the case for a highly complex, high risk client), the Need to Know section can indicate 'See complete Care Plan and/or ask members of the care team.'

Stressor Profile

The Stressor Profile Section identifies the triggers to be avoided. Without this information caregivers are forced to function reactively rather than proactively. If the caregiver is not aware that a client cannot tolerate noise, then there is no preparation or problem solving performed when twenty school children from the intergenerational program visit at 10 AM. Likewise, if a client becomes agitated when near Mary Smith and the only empty chair is next to this lady then the caregiver responsible for this client will only find out after sitting her next to Mrs. Smith. In this case, the Stressor Profile section of the client's Care Plan Summary would indicate:

Stressor Profile: *Identify triggers to be avoided for this client i.e. noise, other clients, etc.*

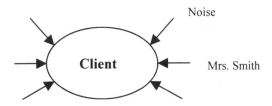

In this way all in contact with the client can be proactive, problem solving what will be done when the children are visiting at 1000 hours or looking for another location to sit the client other than next to Mrs. Smith.

Daily Log

This section of the Care Plan Summary guards the client's ritualistic patterned behavior. The Daily Log section lists where the client should be at what time, doing what.

In one example, the care team who knew the client required a nap each morning for thirty minutes and needed to be awakened before 1030 hours. They discovered that any longer or awakening her any later resulted in the client being too drowsy for lunch. Unfortunately with word-of-mouth communication and difficulty reading all care plans at the beginning of the shift, other caregivers did not know these details. Some were not aware that she had a nap in the morning. Others who knew the client had a nap in the morning would let her sleep longer or arrange the nap time so she was awakened after 1030 AM. They then believed that the problems at lunch was normal for this client.

If the client is always up at 0715 hours and last to the dining room, then that time and routine cannot be changed unless the client demonstrates that the norm is no longer working. The Daily Log section allows all caregivers to personalize the client's day by maintaining ritualistic routines and schedules, inadvertently decreasing stress and lessoning challenging behaviors.

The following is an example of the Daily Log Section for this client:

Daily Log: *Identify exact times for daily routines/schedules*

Time	Routine	Time	Routine
0715	Up, washed and dressed (see base line data)	1030 to 1100	Sits in yellow chair by the window in lounge listening to classical music. Will wander hall and return to chair
0800	Breakfast, last in the dining room	1100 to 1130	Sits at nursing station stapling papers
0830	Toilet (see base line data)	1200	Lunch, last in dining room
0900	Recreational Program if not distressed (see Need to Know and Programming Map)	1245	Toilet (see base line data)
0945 to 1015	Nap		
1015	Toilet (see base line data)		

Need to Know
This section provides the supportive measures necessary to care for the client: what to talk about, what not to discuss, clues indicating distress, distracting tactics, other supportive measures, etc.

The Care Plan Summary provides information that allows all in contact with the client to be client centered, and inadvertently eliminates controllable distressors that will lead to challenging behaviors.

Updated at the care conference or care plan review, the location or locations of the summary sheets depends on the care setting. They can be located on a clip board with all client assignments for that shift; behind the closet door in the client's room; inside the bedside table door; in the bathroom; under the placemat in the dining room; behind the individuals favorite chair; and so on. Do not restrict the summary to one location, the information is too critical to the client to be inaccessible to the caregiver.

Value of the Care Plan Summary
The Care Plan Summary becomes an excellent advocacy tool, providing specific details about the client to anyone in contact with the individual.

- *Reveals secrets* - This form allows all caregivers to replicate the supportive measures for each individual client. It is essential that all caregivers, regardless of their position or function, refer to the Care Plan Summary before initiating any contact with the client.

- *Easily accessible information* - Although detailed care plans are available, the time at the beginning of the shift to read all care plans is limited; access to care plans may be inaccessible to certain individuals (housekeeping, maintenance, volunteers, etc.); and/or the comprehensiveness and details of a complete care plan may make it difficult to decipher what is important. On the other hand, the location or multiple locations of the Care Plan Summary and the brevity of the information provided makes it an excellent reference tool for all.

- *Accountability* - Word-of-mouth communication does not allow for accountability. When a caregiver is challenged for sitting the client next to Mary Smith, the response by the caregiver can be "I didn't know." When the Care Plan

Summary is provided and the client is found sitting next to Mary Smith, the caregiver has only two reasons why this action was taken – she did not refer to the Care Plan Summary or refuses to comply with the required care for this client. In either case the actions of the caregiver can be considered negligent - intentionally ignoring information about a client that results in negative consequences to the individual's safety or well being. A situation where the caregiver must be challenged.

The Care Plan Summary provided is a guideline only. It is important to adapt the information, what is recorded and where it is located to the specific care setting and the needs of the care team.

Success Oriented Charting
Links: Behavioral Incident Assessment, Patterning

One of the most common forms of documentation or charting can be called problem or failure focused charting. Problem or failure focused charting is a description of what was observed. When dealing with medical issues it is highly successful. No analysis is required when describing a wound. However, in behavior management this form of documentation is too limiting. Two flaws exist with problem or failure focused charting:

- *Commonly identifies the problem only* - Frequently when a behavior is elicited from a client, what is charted is simply a description of what was observed i.e. "Became very disruptive, wandering the halls, did not eat supper, did not settle." This provides little information to subsequent caregivers and the care team in general. When this issue is discussed or analyzed at the next care conference, the care team can do little about what is identified unless the individual who charted the behavior is present.

- *Exceptions are often overlooked* - Problem or failure focused charting only addresses concerns or problems. In one case a charting review revealed:

  Monday - "Very disruptive, wandering the halls, did not eat supper, did not settle."
  Tuesday - "Very disruptive, wandering the halls, did not eat supper, did not settle."
  Wednesday - "Very disruptive, wandering the halls, did not eat supper, did not settle."
  Thursday - "Quiet evening"
  Friday - "Very disruptive, wandering the halls, did not eat supper, did not settle."

  This poses a question - What was different about Thursday?

In behavior management a "solution focused" rather than "problem focused" documentation methodology is required. A technique called Success Oriented Charting provides the needed information and ongoing analysis.

Success Oriented Charting requires the caregiver to analyze each behavioral response as it occurs. When staff encounter behavioral outbursts or an intensifying of behavior, it is imperative that they chart more than a description of the problem. Success Oriented charting is a two pronged approach:

- Behavior Present
- Behavior Absent

Behavior Present

In Success Oriented Charting the caregiver must analyze a behavioral outburst when it occurs, identifying what is believed to be causing the behavior and recommending what may be needed to prevent it.

Knowing that all behavior communicates, analyzing the behavior when it occurs provides the care team direction during the subsequent care conference discussions; identifies time and event patterns; and provides recommendations based on the assessment and insights of the caregiver witnessing the behavioral response.

In one situation the documentation during one evening shift utilizing Success Oriented Charting was as follows:

> 1915 hours - Client disruptive in lounge, calling out. Sitting in lounge from supper (1700 hours), TV on for the entire time and other client (Mr. Smith) in lounge also calling out. Recommend programming for this client be initiated at 1800 hours, programming or evening care initiated for Mr. Smith at 1900 hours while this client is in the lounge, and the TV be off with music playing instead or appropriate video tapes provided.

The benefits of the analysis component of Solutions Focused Charting are :

- The information is client specific and solutions oriented.
- The care team receives direction on what may be done differently to change the circumstances leading to the behavioral response.
- Potential triggers have been identified that can be added to the Stressor Profile section of the Care Plan Summary.
- Adaptations to the Daily Log of both this client and Mr. Smith's Care Plan Summary can be made.
- Direction is provided to the entire care team to determine appropriate programming and supportive measures to address the concern.

Behavior Absent

With Success Oriented Charting, the absence of a consistent behavior requires the caregiver to identify what is different about that day, shift or time. Documenting "Quiet evening" is a lost opportunity. Knowing that the mentally impaired communicate by behavior, absence of a consistent behavioral response indicates that something is missing (potential trigger) or that something is different (possible supportive measure) to change the response of the client. In the above case where the client was distressed four of five evenings, it was discovered that on the Thursday evening the TV was broken, the Friday evening it was fixed. Identifying the difference provided significant direction on the supportive measures required for the client in question.

Behavior Analysis is essential to managing any behavior. Utilizing Care Analysis, the Care Plan Summary and Success Oriented Charting allows the care team to determine the specific cause for any behavior, communicate the required supportive measures to all in contact with the client and maintain an ongoing assessment of the results or outcomes experienced.

Chapter Thirteen

Programming

There is a misconception about programming as it applies to the mentally impaired elderly. It is often believed that programming involves recreational activities only. That is not the case. In behavior management programming can incorporate nearly everything that is in contact with the client having direct or indirect positive impact on the client's behavior.

Where assessment determines the need, programming provides the supportive measure required to address the need or manage the behavior. Components of programming that will be discussed in this chapter include:

Benefits
- Goals
- Objectives
- Outcomes

Options (PAA)
- Retract
- Divert
- Redirect

Focus (PAA)
- Client
- Other Clients
- Unit
- Staff

Assessment (PAA)
- Involved/no change
- Involved/Exhausted
- Involved/Excited
- Distressed/Distressed

Opportunities
List of programming that can be employed

Tools
- Programming Map
- Roving
- Layering
- Cloning

PAA indicates that the identified section is detailed in the text Preventing Alzheimer's Aggression. These areas will be summarized in this text to provide a complete overview of programming.

Programming Benefits

The best term to describe programming is opportunity. In one setting a dementia client with repetitive behavior was sitting in the lounge. She continually tore paper, magazines, facial tissue, etc. into little bits. She had piles of little bits on her, on the floor, everywhere. In the other corner was another dementia client who demonstrated rummaging and hoarding behavior. Programming is simple. Direct the individual with rummaging and hoarding behavior to pick up the little bits.

Programming represents the creative side of care (flexibility, consistency, creativity). In one case a wandering client demonstrated rummaging and hoarding behavior that was very disruptive to other clients on the unit. The registered nurse employed an excellent supportive measure. When it was time to dispense medication she gave this client a small paper bag. As the registered nurse toured the unit dispensing medication she would purposely leave medicine cups, bits of paper, etc. on table tops. The client accompanying her was encouraged to pick up the garbage and place it in her paper bag. This lasted 45 minutes. During that time the client enjoyed the task and was not going into the rooms of others.

The goals, objectives and benefits for programming as they apply to Behavior Care are as follows:

Goal: Enhance quality of life.

Objectives:
1) To decrease distress/fear/anxiety.
2) To enhance functioning ability.
3) To individualize approach and care.
4) To reduce the frequency or intensity of challenging behaviors.

Desired Benefits to the Client
- provide purpose
- initiate thought process
- exhaust energy.

There are two forms of programming - add on and add to. The opportunity for add on (additional work over and above what exists) is limited, however "add to" (linked with tasks already being performed) is only as restrictive as the caregiver's creativity. An example of "add on" programming would be scheduling a power walk during a client's high risk times. An example of an "add to" programming is power walking a client when the caregiver walks up and down the hall to transport other clients from the lounge to the dining room.

Programming Options (PAA)

There are three programming options that achieve the programming objectives. Each option creates specific outcomes and each has a number of programming opportunities available that will create that outcome.

Retracting Measures - involves removing the person from a trigger or stressor to let him settle (i.e. being removed from the lounge during a large group activity), or removing the stressor or trigger from the person and let him settle (i.e. relocating another client that is disruptive or turning off the TV). A more descriptive term for retracting measures is to "back off".

Diversional Measures - are used to alter the client's emotional state by changing the individual's thought process. This goes beyond simply initiating diversional tactics. Finding something that simply distracts the client will not necessarily change behavior, i.e. playing music when the individual is aggressive. The individual is still distressed. The most effective diversional measures are related to positive past memories. Playing the right song from 1945, mentioning the daughter's name or discussing flowers are specific to the client. Diversional measures or "hooks" represent a supportive measure that changes the client's thought process which in turn changes the individuals emotional state which will change behavior.

Redirecting Measures - are programs that redirect the client's energy to a more positive outlet. Exhausting the client's energy decreases the intensity, frequency and/or duration of any behavior. Power walks, exercise programs, chores, etc. are valuable and enjoyable to the client, and at the same time decrease the amount of energy available for the behavior.

Programming Focus (PAA)

Programming focus determines the appropriate direction for the supportive measure. This is a sequencing of need that determines the direction for the supportive measures - Client, Other Clients, Unit, and/or the Caregiver.

If the supportive measures decrease the frequency, intensity and/or duration of a client's behavior, then the other clients, the unit in general and the caregivers will also benefit. However, when a client's behavior cannot be managed effectively, i.e. repetitive verbal behavior, then the focus must be on decreasing the impact on the client who is the most sensitive to the repetitive speech (offsetting care and programming schedules), managing the noise level of the unit, and focusing on the tolerance level of the caregiver (limiting contact of any one staff member during each shift).

Programming Assessment (PAA)

When discussing programs it is important to emphasize that the client will indicate the timing and appropriateness.

- Patterning determines when - Programming is not a haphazard schedule of events. Appropriate timing for programming is identified by Patterning (defining the client's time and event patterns). The care team must then determine the appropriate supportive measures that can be implemented prior to those times and/or events in order to break the pattern or remove the person from the potential stressor.

- Trial and error determines what - Appropriateness is based on the concept that "everything works, nothing works". Although certain concerns or negative outcomes can occur with certain activities, some mentally impaired clients may respond positively to those activities. Through trial and error assessment, the client will demonstrate the benefits or value of the programming initiated by his response during or after. If the client becomes distressed during a program then it is obvious the individual cannot tolerate the stimuli as it is presented. However, the second level of assessment is after the program.

There are four possible after responses to program involvement:

- Involved/No Change - The individual is involved and enjoys the program, however the physical, mental and emotional state of the client before the program is the same as after - "right program, right client."

- Involved/Exhausted - The individual is involved and enjoys the program, however the client is exhausted after the program. It is not a problem if the person is allowed to rest or nap. After the rest period the client will return to his normal physical, mental and emotional state.

- Involved/Excited - The individual is involved and enjoys the program, however the client is excited or stimulated by the program. The client needs to walk off the increased energy in order to return to her normal physical, mental and emotional state.

- Distressed/Distressed - The individual is involved and enjoys the program, however the client is highly distressed after the program resulting in high risk behavior; possible risk for the caregiver or others around the individual; and there is a potential need for sedation to settle the person. Programs with this impact are better termed a taboo - the negative consequences outweigh the benefits. How else can the client indicate problems with what is being done until after it is over? His response usually means that the program is too complex or too long and needs to be tailored to the individual's ability, or may indicate that it is inappropriate for this client and should be avoided.

Programming Opportunities

Standing next to a mentally impaired client while he is sitting at the dining room table and asking him to hand over his used glass, plate and utensils is programming. Regardless of how long the task lasts, it gives purpose, exhausts energy and initiates thought process.

It is important when discussing programming opportunities that all potential options be examined regardless of the length of time involved or the simplicity of the task completed. In fact one of the basic concepts for effective programming for the mentally impaired elderly is to keep it simple.

- Simple, regarding what the person is to remember.
- Simple, regarding what the person is asked to do.
- Simple, regarding the instructions given.
- Simple, regarding what is expected of the person.
- Simple, in what will be achieved.

The list of available programming for the mentally impaired is extensive. All activities appropriate for any older adult are appropriate for this clientele, as long as they are adapted to the person's cognitive functioning level, and physical and mental ability. Only some of those will be discussed here.

Ritualistic Activities
Client daily routines and behavioral patterns must be considered when developing programming schedules. It is imperative to incorporate the client's ritualistic activities in the programming schedule, i.e.:

- assisting with chore related activities (cleaning tables, gathering or folding laundry).
- conversing with housekeeping staff while they perform their duties.
- time of favorite TV or radio programs.
- nap, snack or wandering times.

The Programming Map (described later in this chapter) and the Care Plan Summary are useful tools to guard the client's ritualistic pattern. They ensure that more structured programs are not in conflict with these events; provide direction on what other available programs may be appropriate; and outline a complete overview of the client's activity level.

Communication Groups

Communication groups of some type or another seem to be the trend now. Communication or discussion groups may be appropriate for the mentally impaired functioning at level one. However, for many level two mentally impaired clients, communicating for any length of time is a demanding process at a one-to-one level let alone a group setting.

To carry on a conversation it is necessary to concentrate on what was just said, determine what needs to be said in reply and then decide where the conversation is leading - a process that the mentally impaired must find demanding and confusing. During a group discussion it becomes even more complex, a mentally impaired client must:

- concentrate on one person speaking.
- try to understand what that person is saying.
- maintain the train of thought in order to reply.
- suddenly another person speaks.
- quickly identify who it is.
- concentrate on what is being said.
- then another speaks.

The process repeats itself again and again.

Being required to "bounce" from person-to-person in order to keep up with the conversation creates a state of bombarding - over stimulation that will result in the person feeling out of control, becoming increasingly agitated at the demands of the task, or withdrawing from the stimulus experienced.

Too many communication groups result in the group leader (a staff member) talking to one client, then moving to the next, with little or no interaction maintained between clients. The value of such an exercise is questioned. It is better to work with an individual at a time and forget the group, rather than subject the mentally impaired to such a complex task.

This is not to say that communication groups should stop. With anything involving the mentally impaired - if it works, don't change it. Carrying on a conversation where the caregiver is the principal speaker and the client is encouraged to participate when he wishes, seems to be the least demanding for some. If the client participates in any way, or is an active observer, then by all means continue with the group. If any client merely sits there with little or no response, then this may not be the activity for that person. More commonly, a roving communication exercise (described later in this chapter) that lasts only a few moments seems to have the greatest impact.

Sensory Stimulation
Sensory deprivation is a common experience of the mentally impaired. Sensory deprivation occurs when the environment is void of the natural colors, aromas and sensations we are accustomed to experiencing.

The experience of sensory deprivation can be demonstrated well. If a client lounge in a health care facility has vinyl furniture, it is fascinating to watch the response of a mentally impaired client who has the opportunity to sit on a crushed velvet couch. As soon as she makes contact with the fabric, she will continually stroke it. Her behavior demonstrates the intensity of the sensation created by that material. Not experiencing such a sensation for a long time, she finds the sensation very intense and highly stimulating. The fabric creates a heightened sensory stimulation effect. Many substances will create the same effect.

Giving a whole onion and a paring knife to a mentally impaired client will result in the same response. Encouraging her to cut it, feel it and smell it, will often create an obvious reaction. She may even take a bite from it - that will no doubt cause sensory stimulation.

Sensory stimulation involves providing opportunities to experience tactile, auditory, taste, visual and smell sensations. A sensory box containing fabrics, sandpaper, anything that the client has not handled for some time will have a phenomenal impact.

Bringing leaves in during the fall and placing them on a table, or a bucket of snow in the winter and have clients place their hands in them. Spices to smell. Exotic foods to taste. Their reaction will be most rewarding.

Environmental Attractors

Environmental attractors are objects that will attract the mentally impaired and hold their attention for any length of time. There are two excellent examples - museum displays and activity centers.

Museum displays require enclosed glassed cabinets throughout the unit in view of the wandering path (for safety the glass should be removed and replaced with Plexiglas, and the doors locked). The local museum is then asked to supply community related antiques and collectables to place in the cabinets. In one example one of these cabinets was located at the end of the hall. A client who was non-communicative, responded poorly to any structured programming and was a chronic wanderer, would walk up to the cabinet and stare at a small butter churn for three or four minutes, turn and walk down the hall, then return to stare for another three to four minutes. This obviously stimulated a specific past memory and also decreased her wandering behavior by 25%. The contents of the cabinets are replaced every month unless a client relates to a specific item. The museum is then asked if the object can remain in the cabinet.

Activity centers are extremely valuable. They are intended to attract the dementia client to manipulate objects at the center. (*Caution*: it is important that these centers be "mentally impaired proof", securing potential weapons to the desk or table top, ensuring there are no sharp objects, etc.). Activity center examples include:

Office Center - office desk, chair, old adding machine, writing paper, stapler, file folders.

Wedding Center - wedding pictures, gown, flowers.

Sewing Center - cloth measuring tape, comforter secured to a table with buttons, zippers, and tabs attached that can be manipulated but not removed.

Gardening Center - flowers, gardening books.

Carpenter Center - sand paper, wooden blocks, fabric measuring tape, simple ready to assemble wooden projects.

Clients who may have an interest in a specific center should be brought to it frequently to help them become familiar with it.

Music

Music to many older people means more than just entertainment. In fact, prior to the 1950's or the age of television, music was the main source of entertainment, encompassing almost every social event.

What was the top song in 1972?

Most of our generation would not know. Ask an older person the top song during the war and she will probably be able to tell you. That song was heard thousands of times.

Play the "right" old song and certain mentally impaired clients who normally seem incapable of maintaining any conversation or coherent thought, may sing that song from beginning to end without missing a word. That client is probably singing from old memory, virtually back in the 1940's when she heard it so often.

Certain music brings back memories for all of us. A soft, conventional song can elicit a very positive response from many mentally impaired.

Children

Place a baby in the arms of a mentally impaired client and you will probably see a dramatic shift in that person's behavior. It takes considerable memory loss to forget how to respond to a baby or a young child.

A number of facilities have implemented effective children's programs, formally called intergenerational programs. One such program is to have a child daycare center within the facility. Few facilities have the resources to run one of these on their own. What they have done instead is to lease space within the facility to a privately run daycare business. In that way the operation of the daycare center is not the responsibility of the facility, but the clients living in that facility are encouraged to participate through such avenues as the "hug-a-kid program." Many mentally impaired clients respond beautifully to such an opportunity.

Other facilities have linked client programming opportunities with local schools, implementing an "adopt-a-grandparent program." This program encourages individual students or whole classrooms to adopt one client as a "grandparent." The students are then encouraged to visit and send cards on special days. Whenever such a program is implemented, it is important that a representative of the facility present to the students information about the facility, the clients and their needs, so that they are prepared for what they may encounter and what may be asked of them. Likewise, children involved with specific clients need to be buddied with a staff member or volunteer that knows the client, who can act as a resource when the child visits.

Other children programs involve older children who are encouraged to visit to help certain clients during mealtimes. In fact, many high schools have what are called life enrichment credits. These are recognized credited programs where students are allowed to take a certain amount of time each month from school in order to participate in a community based assignment. Assisting on specific units within a facility provides an ideal learning base for some students. Any of these programs are useful on any unit to establish an atmosphere that is normal and healthy.

By the way, the children are usually very receptive when involved with the mentally impaired elderly, as long as they are supported and prepared for what may occur on the unit. In fact, the younger the child, the better the rapport. If any problems do occur, they usually arise from the parents. Stereotypic beliefs about a long term care facility, and those who live within it may limit the open-mindedness of certain parents, which can make such opportunities for the children difficult. It is important before any program is implemented that the parents are helped to understand the purpose and role of the children's visits.

Pets

Many facilities have introduced pets. Fish and birds are probably the most universal, dogs and cats are the up and coming rage. The pet used must be a "people sensitive animal," one that knows who and who not to go to. It must be remembered, that there are many people who normally do not like cats or dogs. Likewise, there are certain mentally impaired clients who cannot tolerate them as well. To have a cat or dog jump on the lap of such a client without warning, will result in the cat or the client being injured. The cat will be injured, when the client grabs it to fling it off his lap. The client will be injured, when he grabs the cat. If the animal cannot effectively determine which client to avoid, then it should not be on the unit.

Some facilities have brought in dogs or cats from the local humane society. In some instances, this has created some difficulties. An animal that may appear friendly when in contact with one person, may not be able to handle a unit with thirty people. One of the best animals to arrange for visitations are those from kennel clubs. These are well trained animals the owners are pleased to display. Another source of pets for visitation is from staff themselves. Encouraging staff to bring in their own pets for the shift they are scheduled is very effective.

Those willing to go "the extra mile" to provide its clients the fullest degree of quality of life are always admired. One facility had an enclosed courtyard. They would periodically put rabbits or a goat in that area. The clients would feed and talk to the animals. It was amazing to watch the response by some.

Bursts of Activity

As identified in our earlier discussion on wandering, it is not uncommon for the mentally impaired to have a poor attention span. Planned bursts of activity are important and must consciously be integrated into the care routine. If energy of the mentally impaired is not exhausted in a conscious effort, then it will impact on the success of any care task as the day progresses.

Activities such as turning on a radio and performing passive exercises with this client, taking one arm and then the other and helping the person raise and lower them, are simple supportive measures. Taking a client or group of clients for a walk, going at a pace and distance that is within the person's physical limit, is another quick option. Encouraging certain clients to follow staff as they conduct rounds or pick up equipment, is always valuable. When implemented on an ongoing and informal basis, they not only release the built up energy of the client, but also provide staff an opportunity to enhance their rapport with those under their care. By the way, the staff who work well with this type of clientele and who understand them, usually undertake such interventions if they are clear that they have the permission to do so.

Activities of Daily Living (ADL)

Integrating certain ADL tasks as programs is also valuable. An effective activity is to help a mentally impaired client shave himself, who has in the past been shaved by staff. This simple task can accomplish a great deal more than mere shaving. Think about it for a moment! What needs to be done to help a client shave himself? The steps would be as follows:

Take the electric razor (turned off) and place it in his hand, then turn it on (sensory stimulation). While the client is sitting in front of the mirror, place one hand on his shoulder and use the other to guide his hand with the razor. Move the razor to his face, identifying where on his face you are touching him, and encouraging him to look in the mirror during the process.

What you have accomplished here is very meaningful.

- Sensory stimulation by feeling the razor on his own face and in his hand.
- Sensory stimulation by touching him as you are doing the process.
- Purposeful hand and arm movement, raising the razor to his face and moving it from one side to the other, a movement he may not have performed for some time.

- Body awareness by identifying left and right side of his face, his chin, etc.

There is a further side benefit to this task. If he is capable of performing this movement on his own, the razor can be replaced with a face cloth or a spoon.

Chores
Many clients will respond better to chores than to most recreational activities. Chores are tasks that the client has performed all of her life. She may no longer be able to perform the task well or even to complete it, but she can still feel useful by attempting it.

When one remembers that our clients have been caregivers all of their lives, not care receivers, it is easy to identify how important chores become. There is a constant need for some mentally impaired clients to do what is familiar and what feels useful. It is not uncommon to see mentally impaired clients wiping table tops, picking up bits of paper or articles of clothing, even helping other clients. Their performance may not be complete or even accurate, but they are often focused on the task for a varying amount of time.

Chores must be integrated into programming. Washing ten medicine cups over and over again, folding a couple of towels, cleaning table tops repeatedly, pushing a broom around, sweeping the same piece of dirt, all have a function. You are aware of the task being repetitive, not the client. If a mentally impaired client was aware that he was completing the same task again and again, it would increase his anxiety and lead to an agitated response. Those who proclaim that a client should not be allowed to do such a repetitive task because it is not normal, have forgotten that expecting "normal" behavior is asking too much of our mentally impaired.

Once again, if I had right sided paralysis from a stroke and could only use my left arm, would you stop me from performing all tasks because I could not do them as a "normal" person? No, you would adjust the task to fit my existing strengths and limitations, praising me for performing to the best of my ability.

If I am mentally impaired, doing that one task over and over again may be my optimum functioning level. No one knows what doing that task means to me. It can provide:

- a sense of purpose
- a feeling of being needed
- active range of motion exercises
- energy release in a positive manner.

It is better to have a client fold a couple of towels for a half an hour, than stare at a blank wall for the same length of time or wander aimlessly through the hall.

Pictorial History
Creating a client pictorial history is a valuable reminiscent tool. Earliest to the most recent photos of a client are placed in a photo album with the year and description of the photo beneath it. This is not something that should be done without the client's participation. Pictures that having meaning for the family may be forgotten by the client. To build the pictorial history, family need to show a series of pictures to their family member. If there is no reaction when the picture is viewed by the client and the situation discussed, then it is not used. If there is any response (increased attentiveness, changes in facial expression, comments of any type, etc.) then it is placed in the album in chronological order. Anyone in contact with the client can then use the pictorial history to initiate a very specific client centered conversation about meaningful past events.

Doing Something "Crazy"
One of the qualities demonstrated by effective caregivers is the ability to periodically do something a bit "crazy." No routine or schedule is set in stone. Caregivers in a health care organization need to be told that they can go anywhere they want during their work day, as long as they take their clients with them. This freedom to break the routine is an effective means to give staff the permission to be

flexible. Taking the clients on a picnic or to the zoo provides an atmosphere of normalcy.

An integral and rewarding part of our job is to have "fun." If caregivers enjoy themselves, the clients are probably having a good time as well.

Expanding Staff Contact
The following is a comment that usually raises some eyebrows -

> *It is important that staff from any department be allowed the freedom to stop at any time during their shift for a break or a cup of coffee, as long as they are having it with two clients who are mentally impaired.*

This opportunity requires an environment that trusts its staff (to allow the freedom), but also one that maintains accountability for job performance (to prevent any abuse of that freedom).

There is an endless list of activities in which the mentally impaired can participate. To make any activity successful requires creativity. To do or try things that others may have trouble relating to, but are usually very effective, separates those caregivers who work well with the mentally impaired, from those who do not.

Programming Tools

In health care organizations, the coordination of programming is a challenge. Knowing who is doing what when for each individual client is no easy task. The following tools expand programming usage and enhance communication:

Programming Map
Programming Drawer
Roving
Layering

It is important to emphasize that these tools are not for recreation purpose, but effective behavior care practices. Recreation staff have the ability to enhance and expand what is described, and may even have alternatives that achieve the results.

These practices are provided as general guidelines as they apply to behavior care practices, the care team is encouraged to adapt these tools to fit the specific needs within their setting.

Programming Map

Programming can often encounter specific challenges. It is common to witness programming conflicts amongst caregivers. Programming conflicts occur when caregivers inadvertently or unwittingly:

- schedule a program in conflict with another.
- schedule multiple programs in succession overwhelming the client.
- initiate programs that are not known to the rest of the care team.
- do not know that a program is available or scheduled where a specific client could participate.
- do not know the client's involvement in a specific program that could be initiated when the client is distressed.

Examples of programming conflicts are many. In one care facility, while a recreation staff member did her rounds of the unit, she would visit a specific client if found sitting in her normal spot by the door. However, the rest of the care team did not know about this or if it was known, there was no formal tool to communicate it to others (other than word-of-mouth communication). It was common for nursing staff to schedule this client's morning care at the same time as recreation was touring the unit. Not only was the opportunity lost on many occasions, but the sporadic contact limited the recreation staff member's ability to deepen the contact. Had the contact been consistent each morning, the recreation staff member would have invariably brought along specific objects to discuss or treats to eat that would make the visits even more meaningful.

The same can occur with structured recreation activities. Recreation may inadvertently schedule a client for a recreational activity in the morning not knowing that at the same time the housekeeper would have carried on a conversation with the client each morning while she cleans her room or that nursing staff have the client pick up garbage or linen at that time. Our resources are too limited and the client's needs too great to lose these opportunities.

A Programming Map coordinates programming to ensure the right program at the right time. A Programming Map involves the following (see sample next page):

- all available programming for the unit or facility are listed at the top of a flip chart sheet or bristle board (ideally this is developed utilizing a computer). This includes those conducted by recreation staff as well as others (direct care staff, volunteers, family members).
- on the left column is the list of client names.
- the following code is used under each programming item:
  - (√) indicates that the client is involved in this program.
  - (X) indicates that this program has been deemed inappropriate for this client.
  - (O) indicates that it is not known if this program is appropriate and needs to be assessed.
- next to each (√) is the time and days of the week the client is involved in that program.

The programming Map is valuable for all caregivers; should be located where it is visible to the care team; and discussed and updated at the care conference.

Programming Map

Name	Family Visit	Department Visit	Chores	Power Walk	Exercise	Baking	Reminiscing
Hilda Smith	√ M, W 1400	√ M to S HK 1000	√ M to Su N 0830	X	X	√ F 1400	√ T, Th, S, Su V 1400
George Doe	X	X	X	M to Su N 0900, 1100, 1400, 1700	O M to F 1300	X	O S, Su V 1300
Alice Dupelli	√ M to F 1000	√ M to F R 0830	√ M to Su D 1130	X	X	O F 1400	X
Mohamid Ba	√ Su 1300	O T Mn 1300	O T Mn 1300	√ M,W,F N 1500	√ M to S 1430	√ F 1400	

√ - involved	P - Porters	M - Monday	F - Friday
O - being assessed	SU - Sets-up	T - Tuesday	S - Saturday
X - not involved	C - Cleans	W - Wednesday	Su - Sunday
R - Roving Prog		Th - Thursday	

N - Nursing	D - Dietary
V - Volunteer	Fm - Family
HK - Housekeeping	
Mn - Maintenance	

A Programming Map provides many benefits, it:

- monitors the involvement of all clients in programming (indicated by the number of √'s)
- identifies all available programs in the client programming record (see Programming Drawer).
- indicates when certain programs should be deleted from the programming schedule (specific activity programs where there are few √'s and many X's).
- provides direction to develop new programs as client needs and abilities change (clients who have few √'s and many X's).
- identifies when a client is being assessed, requiring evaluation of the client's physical, mental and emotional state after the program (indicated by an O).
- identifies all of the clients involved in a program and when (indicated by the number of √'s).
- allows all caregivers to know all available programs (as listed on the Programming Map) to determine if a client should be assessed.
- prevents scheduling conflicts so that the client benefits from all programming opportunities.
- provides direction on what programming options for each client are available to intervene on behaviors (indicated by the number of √'s).
- allows the care team to monitor that the scheduling of programs matches the client's time or event patterns, and ritualistic behavior.

When a client has minimal check marks (√) on the Programming Map, it indicates that what exists does not match the profile or abilities of that individual. This requires the care team to investigate other programming options (utilizing related texts and journals, the Alzheimer's Society, the internet, or contacting programming staff in other health care organizations). Once the new programming opportunity is developed, then other clients within that setting can also be assessed to determine if the new program applies to them. This is an excellent way to continually expand the programming envelope to keep pace with the increasing levels of care.

Roving and Layered Programs

It is obvious that programs lasting longer than 10 to 15 minutes are not appropriate for the majority of mentally impaired clients. Likewise, large group programming (more than 4) has minimal benefits to this clientele. However, shorter (two to four minutes) one-to-one programming will apply to the majority of mentally impaired.

Roving programming is taking whatever program is planned (i.e. sensory stimulation, current event discussion, etc.) and walking it throughout the unit. Each roving program lasts two to four minutes with clients sitting throughout the unit who would not normally be involved. Roving programs are added to the Programming Map (indicated as an R) and Care Plan Summary (Daily Log Section) signaling the client's involvement to other caregivers, encouraging that the client be available to participate.

Layering Programs involves taking one program and breaking it down into specific components, then defining which client(s) can be involved in each component, an example is baking:

- One client is involved in portering.
- A different client involved in the set-up.
- Two different clients involved with the mixing.
- Three others participate in the baking.
- Twelve enjoy the eating of the finished product.
- The first client back again to assist with the portering.
- The second client assists with the clean-up.

One program now has seven layers, where different clients may be involved in one or more of those layers. The times each client is involved is identified on the Programming Map.

Programming Drawer

Recreation staff have the opportunity for more concentrated contact with clients for an extended period of time than any other department. Too often, information gained about a client by the recreation department does not become a part of the care plan or formally shared with the care team. This information can provide other caregivers with significant direction on behavior care practices employed with each client when behaviors are eminent.

The recreation staff are the programming specialists. Their skill set, experience and job responsibilities require them to develop many of the programming opportunities for specific clients. However, that does not mean they are the only ones to conduct them. All caregivers may know the programs a client participates in, however, not all know how to make them functional. The problem in most care settings is that the recreation staff are often the only ones who know specifically the set up, how to motivate, what length of time a client should be involved, the cues to respond to, etc. for the majority of clients on the unit. When the recreation staff leave, they can inadvertently take their program knowledge with them. This leaves other caregivers with the opportunity to conduct programming but not the knowledge on how to do it with a specific individual.

In order to promote others to integrate specific client centered programming into the care routine, it is encouraged that client Programming Drawers be available. These Programming Drawers can be located in a drawer in the client's bedside table or built specifically for all clients in a storage or supply room. A client Programming Drawer contains:

- a list of all programs applicable for this client.
- guidelines on the set-up for each program including:
    - how each program is set-up for individual clients.
    - how the client is encouraged to become involved.
    - the length of time the client normally participates.
    - the response that can be expected.
    - ways to encourage the client to participate.

- results gained from programming involvement .
- related equipment/supplies to conduct the program (i.e. audiotapes, cards, nature book, etc.)

The Program Drawer is valuable for all caregivers, including family members and volunteers. The Program Drawer:

- allows others to replicate the practices of recreation staff.
- initiate a program as required regardless of recreation staff availability.
- provides information to the care team that may be valuable in other care settings.
- allow those with intimate knowledge about the client to provide specific direction on how to enhance further the efforts of recreation.
- provides supportive measure opportunities when a client becomes distressed or needs to be occupied.

What to Say

Anger, frustration, anxiety, depression, sensitivity, elation, excitement, exhilaration, frivolity, all are major components of the human psyche. Each in varying degrees will influence a person's perception, reaction, ability and state of mind.

There is little we know about the link of cognitive ability and emotions. They are not separate entities, but intertwined to affect each other equally. To believe a person in a level two state of functioning cannot experience a variety and range of emotional responses because of memory loss is too simplistic.

The mentally impaired respond to the world around them, as <u>they</u> perceive it. Their ability to appropriately interpret cues and information may be limited, but the range of emotions available to them is still present. In fact, even though a person may have a flat affect, unable to express emotions, it does not mean that emotions are not felt. There is no question that as the disease progresses some emotions may be lost, some may become distorted and exaggerated, some over powering and ever present.

The challenge to the caregiver is to understand the impact of emotions in association with mental impairment. The mentally impaired respond in a personalized, reactionary manner - identifying a few bits of information from a given situation, interpreting it within their mental time frame and limited mental abilities, and then reacting in the manner available to them. The more we can understand their perceptions, the more effective our interventions and supports.

What To Say is one of the most common questions asked by caregivers. Before discussing this topic, it is important to compare its length to the rest of the book. This section on what to say to the mentally impaired will only encompass a couple of pages. Our discussion on the other options of care requires substantially more time and space.

A verbal response to a mentally impaired client has minimal sustained impact for a number of reasons.

1) The client's poor memory retention and comprehension skills make what we say only a temporary supportive measure. Anything that is said to a mentally impaired client is often forgotten as soon as it is heard.

2) We have already established that the world of the mentally impaired is very real to them. Continually contradicting or correcting strips away from that client what he believes is right, and may create further confusion or even an agitated response.

It is more important that we invest our energies and resources into developing effective and flexible care practices, than to concentrate excess energy on the skill of what to say. It is the environment, the care routines, approach, assessment tools, concepts, etc. that will have a more sustainable impact on this client than anything else. If they are not adequately developed, nothing we say will compensate for their absence.

There is no magic statement that will stop the repetitive demands or questions of the mentally impaired. In fact the past practice of Reality Orientation or repeatedly correcting the mentally impaired does not work. It does nothing to change the client's perception of what is happening. Bluntly correcting the client with no sensitivity to what he is experiencing is in essence saying to the mentally impaired, "You are wrong." That limited response only strips away the client's reality (how he sees it), when he cannot relate to our reality (how we see it), therefore leaving him with nothing. His only response is to become more confused or agitated due to the intensified anxiety created.

Imagine that you believed that someone had just stolen an article of your clothing. You would be upset. To tell you, "No one has stolen your clothing", does not stop the anger you are experiencing. The same is true with the mentally impaired client who believes that someone stole her clothing. She is angry. Telling her she was wrong does nothing about the emotions she is feeling.

Caregivers, who work "magic" - who are successful with certain mentally impaired clients, when others are not - are successful because they take that person seriously. Regardless of the content of what the client is saying, the emotions surrounding it are real. The emotions are not dissolved by just telling the person she is wrong.

In order to respond to the question of what to say to a mentally impaired client, we must return to the first chapters of this book. We began this text with a discussion about the importance of seeing the situation as the mentally impaired client sees it. The more we can understand what the client is experiencing, the more accurately we can adjust our approach.

Likewise, we have emphasized frequently that there can never be only <u>one way</u> to deal with any behavior of the mentally impaired elderly. There are no two clients who are the same, there can be no universal response to fit all. The same is true in what to say, caregivers cannot be limited to only one response. What must be used when communicating to the mentally impaired is a Supportive Approach, one that provides three possible responses:

> "If I believed _____, I would feel _____ as well,
> then . . ." - divert, correct or reminisce.

The first part of this response reinforces how the client sees it and the emotions that experience can elicit. The second part of the response - divert, correct or reminisce, provides options in how to respond.

Diverting is an attempt to get the client's mind off of what he is looking for or what is disturbing him. This is an effective intervention at times. By steering him to something else, he will forget what he was saying, only to return to it once the diversional activity is completed. The Supportive Therapy response in the above example would be:

> "If I believed someone was stealing my clothes, I'd be angry
> as well. Let's sit down and have a cup of coffee (or come help
> me to gather the laundry)."

This approach simply distracts the client. The effect temporarily decreases her agitation and momentarily stops her repetition. As soon as the client has left the diversional activity and stepped into the hallway, she will probably begin again, "They are stealing my clothes, . . ."

A second option is to correct. At times, giving a mentally impaired client the information that is lacking may be appropriate. This manner corrects with a little more compassion.

> "If I believed someone was stealing my clothes, I'd be angry as
> well, but your clothes were dirty and need to be washed. Let me
> take you to the dirty utility room and I will show you where they
> are."

A slight reminder or simple clarification for some mentally impaired is all that is needed. The client may respond, "Oh, that's nice, thank you." Only minutes later it will soon be forgotten and she will return to the hallway, pounding her fist stating, "They are stealing my clothes, . . ."

The third option is to reminisce or talk about what the client is saying. We often forget that we can still speak to a mentally impaired client about the problem without having to correct the content.

Take another example to demonstrate how the Supportive Approach can be utilized. A client says to you, "The baby is hurt. The baby is hurt. . . ." Simply place yourself in that person's situation. Right now you believe a baby has been hurt, how would you feel? The response in return would be:

"If I believed a baby was hurt, I'd be worried too . . ."

You now have three possible responses to complete that sentence:

1. Divert - steer the client to something that will temporarily get her mind off of "the baby."
2. Correct - "I can understand how you believe that there may be a baby crying, it is Mrs. Smith in the next room calling out, let me show you."
3. Reminisce - "I bet you have taken care of many babies, tell me about them."

The tactic used depends on the client's response. If correcting creates further agitation or confusion, then divert or reminisce. If the client becomes agitated when diverted, then reminiscing or correcting become the avenues to take. If reminiscing creates distress, then diversion becomes the only option.

No matter what is said, the client's concern, questions or needs will be expressed again and again (like a scratched record with the needle caught at the same place, replaying itself over and over again). The only salvation, if you consider it as that, is time. As the disease worsens, the memory or awareness of that event or issue will pass. All we can do in the interim is to be supportive, assisting the client with what he is experiencing to the best of our ability.

Understanding Our Limits
A male mentally impaired client

In his late seventies
Is living in your facility./
His wife died two years before admission./
When you sit him at his table for a meal
He exclaims, "Set another place for my wife please, she will
    be here soon."/
Whenever you put him to bed he always asks,
"Would you leave the light on for my wife, she will be
    coming to bed soon."/
Frequently when you meet him in the hall
He will stop you and ask, "Have you seen my wife, I think
    she has gone shopping?"/

The mentally impaired will recall memories that have attached to them intense emotions, either positive or negative. Each time the memory is recalled, those emotions will follow. Be comfortable with the emotions expressed by your mentally impaired clients, whether they evoke tears or anger. You will experience them frequently.

In fact, family will often say - "I don't like talking to Dad about the past, I feel it will make him worse." They believe that because their father cries or gets angry, they have done something wrong. On the contrary, if you don't talk to him about his past, what else do you talk to him about? All he has left is the past.

In John's case, the next response to his question should have been - "John tell me about your wife, she must have been an important part of your life." That response doesn't resolve his emotions nor prevent him from asking about his wife only minutes later. It did allow him to talk about an important part of himself, a major component at that moment for his quality of life.

The Taboos of "What to Say"

There are two things that can be detrimental to the mentally impaired - to lie or to delve further. Imagine, you have an 84 year old mentally impaired client, who repeatedly asks, "Where is my mother?" Some caregivers respond, "Don't worry dear, your mother will be here in a half an hour." In actual fact, her mother died thirty years ago. If you asked the reason for their lie, they will usually state, "It is to keep her quiet." Generally, those are the same caregivers who will sedate or restrain that person, in order to accomplish that one, primary mandate - keep her quiet.

Lying reinforces the client's perception of reality. Those who think it is the best intervention have not looked closely enough at the potential long term consequences. Such a response may quiet the client temporarily. Over the long term it could create more difficult problems to resolve. Reinforcing that client's reality will only intensify her past orientation, increasing her confusion. You have conditioned the client to focus on something that she can easily recall. She will go from asking once every hour, to potentially every five minutes.

The other taboo in communicating with the mentally impaired is to delve further (unfortunately this is becoming a popular trend employed by some). Delving further into what a mentally impaired client says is the same principle employed while counseling. The counselor's responsibility is to uncover the client's problem. To accomplish that goal, the client is forced to define or detail every word or statement. The more details that are added, the better the problem will be understood. Let me demonstrate.

Imagine:

> You are cognitively well.
> You feel your world is "closing in on you." /
> The stress and emotional pressure you are experiencing
> Makes you feel as though you are out of control./
> You come to me for counseling./
>
> I ask, "What is your problem?"
> You respond, "I really don't know what it is.
> All I know is that nothing is going right."/
> "What do you mean nothing is right?"
> "My husband is driving me crazy"
> "What is it about your husband that affects you that way?"

> With each statement you make
> You are required to provide specifics./
> The problem will eventually be uncovered./
> At that moment
> You will experience intense emotions
> Either anger or tears./
> Once those emotions are expressed
> I can then help you
> To learn how to solve your problem./

There is a technique that professes to be an effective way to converse with the mentally impaired elderly. It encourages making the mentally impaired define every word and phrase in order to uncover the true meaning of what the client is saying. The goal is to uncover the real problem. There is no question that a mentally impaired client may be able to respond to that mode of questioning. It is very likely that the conversation would focus the client more on what is bothering him. It is also likely that when that problem is detailed further, you will also stir within that client very intense emotions, either anger or tears. Now what do you do?

> You cannot teach this individual how to resolve what is bothering him.

He will forget any instructions or skills you give him. What is more important is the residual impact of such an approach. When you leave, he will have forgotten what was discussed, but will retain the emotions stirred. What has been the benefit of the time and energy invested? Such an approach is often fruitless and stacked with potential problems.

Caregivers will ask, "How do you deal with a client who continually asks 'Where is my mother?', when you are in her room doing her care for twenty minutes?" The best response:

"If I hadn't seen my mother for a long time, I would really miss her. Tell me what your mother was like"

It is easier to listen to the client talk about her mother (reminisce) than to hear her ask continually where her mother is.

There is no need to go any deeper in discussing the feelings she is experiencing by the loss of her mother, it will not help. Just carry on a normal conversation as you would with anyone else who was interested in talking about her mother. The only difference in the conversation between the client and yourself is the grammatical tense that is used.

The client will talk in the present tense, you need to talk in the past tense. When the client says, "I would like you to meet my mother." Your response should be, "I wish I could have met your mom, I bet she was a very nice person." Again it is subtle, but to argue will only create agitation, to go any deeper will create distress and to lie will only cause further confusion. What is left is to be supportive.

For those who would like things neatly packaged that is frustrating, they see the challenges presented by the mentally impaired as problems that must be resolved, not realities that they must learn to live with. In fact those are often the caregivers who have the greatest difficulty with this clientele.

Others find the challenges created by the mentally impaired as exciting. They know that with this clientele you need to constantly be thinking, constantly creative, and fully involved in what you do. Those who thrive on "the challenge" are the ones who provide to this clientele the greatest level of quality of life possible, given their limitations and strengths. Those caregivers are always impressive to watch in action.

Regardless of the caregiver, there is one fact that remains - to be effective requires a supportive work setting. Such a setting must encourage flexibility and creativity. It must support those who are successful with the mentally impaired and instill in others the same drive and insights.

Chapter Fourteen

The Environment

The environment, if adapted effectively, can be a functional mechanism allowing even a severely impaired client a considerable degree of independence.

The goal in arranging the environment is to keep it as simple as possible, leaving as little to memory as necessary. A process of multiple cueing, having a number of mechanisms to reinforce for this person the needed information, is the most effective approach. The more cueing that can be employed, the better the chance many clients will relate to at least one, enhancing their ability to function, decreasing the anxiety experienced.

There are two overall themes to the supportive measures created when adapting the environment for the mentally impaired with challenging behaviors:

- *making the environment "mentally impaired proof."*
- *keeping it "simple/complicated."*

Making it *mentally impaired proof* is in keeping with the primary philosophy of behavior management - removing the factors that further complicate the person's life. When a client responds to the environment in a way that is detrimental to his well being or the well being of others, the question is not, "How do you stop the client?," but "How do you adapt the environment so the client will not respond in that manner?"

For example, if an exit door can be opened, a dementia client will leave through that door regardless of the weather or risk factor. The client does not have the cognitive ability to identify safety risk and will not remember if told. However, making the door *mentally impaired proof* or securing the door so the client cannot open it removes the safety risk.

The second concept of keeping it *simple/complicated* demonstrates that simple tactics are often all that is needed. A locked door is not required to keep a dementia client from leaving. A numeric key pad controlling a magnetic locking system is all that is needed. Anyone who can operate the numeric key pad can open the door. The dementia client does not have the analytical ability and memory retention to operate the key pad. Making it simple/complicated has secured the door.

The need to adapt the environment was demonstrated well by the following case study. In one facility a level two mentally impaired client was walking down the hall. She peered into a bedroom. The bed by the door had a pulsating mattress on top. On the floor, at the foot of the bed and in plain view was an air pump, with a light that blinked off and on. The wandering client saw the light on the pump. She was attracted to it (*if the stimuli is too intense some cannot help but respond*). She picked up the pump and started walking away with it. Of course it was still connected to the mattress and plugged into the wall. The mattress came with her, and the plug was disconnected. As she headed for the door with her bounty, she bumped into a twenty-nine inch TV on coasters sitting against the wall. That moved, so she took it with her as well.

Staff wanted to stop the client's behavior. There is no way to stop her behavior other than restraining her to a chair or locking all bedroom doors to keep this one client out of those rooms. Both of these dramatic interventions will be ineffectual. The challenge is to adapt the environment to manage her behavior. In this case:

- the pump was placed in a wood box with a lid to hide the light.
- the box was placed under the bed out of view.
- the wheels from the TV stand were removed so that it would be too heavy to move.

Making the environment mentally impaired proof and using simple/complicated strategies allowed the client to wander safely without being drawn to these objects.

Adapting the environment for the dementia client is not as straight-forward as other concepts discussed. Utilizing the majority of supportive measures discussed in this text, i.e. Care Analysis or implementing certain programming options, vary somewhat from location to location, but the general methodology remains intact.

However, the challenge facing environmental supportive measures is to determine how to implement the concepts when no two locations are the same. Not only are the requirements for long term care, acute care, community care and family different. No two long term care facilities are the same in their design, physical layout, etc., just as no two houses are the same in their design, furnishings, lighting, etc.

There are certain environmental measures that are universal regardless of the location. Others are site specific. Site specific environmental challenges tap the creativity of the care team.

The Second Time Factor

A dementia client continually communicates by their behavior. The *second time factor* allows the client to teach us what environmental changes are required. The second time factor is simple:

- First Time - if a dementia client responds to an environmental issue once (other than a safety issue), then little or no action may be required. For example, if the female client went into the bedroom and walked away with the pulsating mattress and TV the first time, then no steps would be taken after the items were returned to the room. Initiating an environmental change to every <u>one time occurrence</u> (other than a safety issue) is costly and often unnecessary.

- Second Time - if a client repeats the same behavior a second time, she has demonstrated the pattern of her behavior which requires steps to be taken to adapt the environment to break that pattern. In this case, not responding to the repeated actions of a dementia client can be costly - increased safety risk, disruptive to others, potential aggressive response when continually corrected or the object is taken away, etc.

To not take action when the client repeatedly demonstrates that an environmental issue creates difficulty is to ignore what she is communicating. The Second Time Factor should be an expected practice for any care team, a philosophy that a client should not be subjected to a negative stimuli more than twice.

Environmental Cueing Options

Environmental cueing is a physical attractor involving an object or color that will draw a dementia client to a specific location. The need for such cueing was emphasized by a mentally impaired client of one facility (as always, it is the client who will teach us the supportive measures required). This gentleman found a magic marker, and proceeded to create a trail to follow. He placed "X" markings on the hallway wall from the lounge to the door of his room. With those markings, he was able to find his room.

The caregivers left the markings on the wall for as long as he could use them. They knew that if he needed them, they were important. They fought off many demands to paint that wall by those who did not understand its importance. Their commitment to the philosophy they professed - Quality of Life for their clients, outweighed any need to aesthetically improve the looks of that wall.

Examples of environmental cues are as follows:

1) Color Coded Door Frames
Painting bedroom doors a different color than the hallway walls is common on units housing dementia clients. However, painting only

bedroom doors a different color is of little value to mentally impaired clients. Bedroom doors are usually left open during the day and are only visible when one is standing in front of them. Painting the door frames along with the doors is of more value. The door frames can be seen no matter where one is standing in the hall.

Painting the door frames different accent colors - red, green, blue, yellow, etc. may be difficult to color coordinate aesthetically, but can be of a functional benefit to the mentally impaired. [Caution - pastel blues or greens, tend to wash out to yellow or gray for some older people due to normal aging changes of the eye - bright blues and greens may be seen clearly.]

A red door frame can easily be spotted from anywhere in the hall. There may be more than one red door frame, but when three or four different accent colors are used, the number of doors to choose from has been decreased dramatically.

Some facilities have taken a middle of the road approach to painting door frames. Rather than painting bedroom doors and door frames one of four different accent colors, only one accent color is used, i.e. a bright blue. One of four different colored square pieces of plexi-glass (approximately 18" x 18") is then placed next to each door frame (client name bar and picture are placed on the plexi-glass, see below).

Before a client is encouraged to find her room by looking for the red door frame or plexi-glass, it is necessary to determine if she can identify the color red. Large sample paint chips (at least 3" x 5" in size) identical to the colors used on the door frames must be available for assessment purposes. Placing the paint chips in a row in front of the client and asking her to pick the red one will determine her ability to identify that color. If she cannot recognize red from the paint chips in front of her, she will be unable to pick the red door frame when walking down the hall. If she can identify the color, it is imperative that she always be directed to her room by saying, "Find the red door frame and you'll find your room."

The client may end up looking into all of the rooms with a red door frame until she finds her belongings or articles. The amount of stimuli to sort through has been decreased. If there are ten bedroom doors in the hall and four colors used, only two or three will be red.

This same concept can be reversed to prevent dementia clients from wandering into rooms that are unsafe (i.e. utility room, housekeeper's closet, etc.). To decrease the amount of wandering into non-client areas the doors and door frames need to be painted the same color of the wall. This camouflaging effect will virtually make these doors disappear from view (if the stimulus is not intense enough, it will be missed or misinterpreted) decreasing the draw for the wandering client to investigate. Having non-client doors and door frames painted the same color as the wall not only removes these doors from sight, but also decreases the number of doors to choose from, making bedroom doors painted a bright color stand out.

2) Name Bars
Name bars are also valuable locator devices. The name bars must be 3 inches (7.5 cm) by 18 inches (45 cm). A name bar that is 1 inch (2.5 cm) by 3 inches (7.5 cm) cannot be seen.

Placing the name bar on a contrasting color plate that matches the color of the bedroom door and frame helps it to stand out - i.e. black and white name bar on a red plastic background, same color as the door frame. The lettering on the name bar must be simple. Fancy script lettering may be attractive, but it is difficult for the mentally impaired to read.

The name used on the name plate must be one that the client can relate to. In one setting, an 82 year old client's name bar read Mr. R. Buckman, however the client related only to Bucky Buckman. Mr. R. means nothing to the mentally impaired. It requires high cognitive ability to be able to interpret letters to mean words. Besides this man had been Bucky Buckman for 82 years of his life.

Before a client is directed to their room by looking for her name, it must be assessed if the person is capable of reading her name. Four dummy name bars are required. The four dummy name bars and the client's name bar is placed in front of the client and the client is asked to pick out her name. If she is unable to identify her name from the five in front of her, she will be unable to identify her name on the wall outside her door.

Remember to lessen the stimuli. If the person can only relate to her first name, then the name bar on her door frame should only have her first name on it. The more clutter, the less able a dementia client is to identify the usable information.

3) Client's Picture

Having the client's picture above or below his name bar may also be of assistance. If there is a concern that the pictures may be easily torn off the wall, Plexiglas covers can be placed over them and bolted to the wall.

Before using the client's picture as a cue to find his room, it is necessary to determine if the client can recognize himself. A client who is 84 years old in the picture, but believes he is 42 in his mind, may not know who he is looking at.

Place five pictures in front of the client, one of him and one of four others. Then ask him to pick out his picture. If he can't pick it out when it is in front of him, he will be unable to pick it out when it is on the wall outside his room.

There is no need to place a client's picture on the door frame if that person is unable to identify it and use it to find his room. The only door frames that should have pictures are those door frames of clients who can use them. Having twenty-five pictures on the wall next to door frames when only five clients are able to relate to pictures only clutters the unit and makes it difficult for those five clients to find their picture. When pictures are on the door frames of those five clients only, it eliminates the amount of information those clients must sort. This fulfills the goal of simplifying the unit.

4) Identifying Décor/Shadow Boxes

For those clients who cannot relate to the colored door frames, name bars or picture, then a fourth option may be available. Having a decoration on the bedroom door that is not duplicated on any other door is of help to some. Installing a shadow box in the wall next to the door frame is another option. Shadow boxes are small cabinets recessed into the wall next to the bedroom. They have a clear plexi-glass door with some type of locking device. Personalized objects can then be placed in the shadow box to attract the client to her room.

The decoration on the door or objects in the shadow box need to be something very specific to this client, usually an object or picture of something in her past. For example, a bell on the door of a client whose name was Mrs. Bell, a bank poster on the door of a client who was a bank manager, etc. Assessing that the client can relate to the object as being her own is a must before any locator object is used.

By the way, none of the environmental cues mentioned above work for every mentally impaired client who is unable to find his room. If ten percent who cannot find their room will be able to relate to the colored door frames, another ten percent to the name bar, another ten percent to their picture and another ten percent to the individualized decor. How does that help? It is simple.

If ten clients cannot find their room when these supportive measures are not in place, only six clients will be unable to find their room when they are in place. It is better to have six dementia clients wandering looking for their room than ten.

These locator devices are valuable for acute care and for the client who lives in the community. Painting the door frames may not be an option, however, name bar, picture and/or décor on the client's bedroom door will help the client find their room and the need to search.

Personalizing The Room

Whatever assists the client in finding her room (color, name bar, picture, or decor) can also be used to assist the client to identify her bed (important in a semi-private or ward room). If a cueing device works in one setting, the goal is to use it for other settings as well. Placing the name bar, color plate, picture or decoration on the footboard of the bed may decrease rummaging behavior by some clients.

A bulletin board at the head of the bed and to the side is of further help. It is the ideal location for family pictures, greeting or birthday cards, etc. Seeing these articles assists some in knowing they are in the right room, at the right bed. A word of caution. Plastic tacks should be avoided. Dementia clients can easily mistake the colored plastic tack as something that can be ingested. Securing pictures to bulletin boards using Velcro is much safer. Small round Velcro pieces are available, one side attaches to the bulletin board, the other side to the picture.

A personal bedspread brought from home (previously described as an anchor - using one object to identify where you are) helps some mentally impaired to find their room. For those clients who have not brought a bedspread from home, ask a major retail outlet to bring in a number of bedspreads with different colors and patterns. Place the spreads in the lounge or auditorium, then allow a few of the mentally impaired clients at a time to scan the spreads until they pick one (remember not all will be able to pick one). Those who are able to pick a specific spread are usually able to do so because the color or pattern stands out for that person (the stimuli is intense). That spread can now be purchased through the client's trust account and placed on her bed. It may now become a significant aid to help that person find her room.

Remember that even though some clients are able to pick out a specific spread in one location once, it does not mean that all will be able to pick out the same spread when it is placed on their bed. You will not know a client's ability to use the spread as an anchor until you try it (a process of trial and error).

Calendars and Clocks

As mentioned earlier, a clock to some mentally impaired clients is meaningless. A large clock in the room at eye level may be of value to some, but the ability of the client must be assessed before the device is used. An old fashioned pendulum chime clock located in the lounge may be the most valuable time piece. It is not intended to help clients to know the time, but rather to hook old memory. It is interesting to see the response of some clients when they hear the chimes.

Knowing the day of the week is of little importance to a mentally impaired client - if I forget it is my bath day, you will remind me. Placing a large bank calendar on the bulletin board in the client's room is not for the client, but more for his family and the staff.

If family visited at 1400 hours and left at 1445 hours, would the afternoon staff be told at report that they were just in? Probably not. Not unless the visit was unusual in some way. If at 1600 hours the client says to one of the afternoon staff, "My family doesn't visit me", what is their response? Not knowing that the family was just in, their only response can be, "They will be in soon!" They were just in less then two hours before, but the staff member is unable to reinforce it.

The purpose of the calendar is for family to record their visits. If the daughter visited at 1400 hours, she is encouraged to write on the calendar the time she was in, how long she stayed and what she discussed or did. If she knows when she plans to visit next, she is encouraged to record that time on the calendar.

Now, when staff hear, "My family never visits," they need only to take the client to the calendar showing when the daughter was last in, how many times she has been in over the last few weeks, and when she plans to visit again. The information may be lost as soon as it is given to the client, but at least caregivers are equipped with an appropriate response specific to that person.

Having family record their visits is also an effective assessment tool. On admission, one of the questions asked of family is, "How often do you plan to visit?" If they expect to visit every second day, but the calendar shows that they have only been in twice in the last two weeks, then the care team has an opportunity to intervene on a potential problem. Without the calendar, it would be difficult to know that a possible problem exists until it is well advanced and possibly too difficult to resolve.

The calendar can communicate very important personal information as well - birthdays (self and family members), anniversaries, etc. This way caregivers can talk with any client about those events while performing care, reinforcing the event as well as the passage of time.

Locator Signs

What is in the client's closet or bedside table? If the only way to know is by memory, then the mentally impaired are lost.

Locator signs can assist some mentally impaired clients to find things in their room. Placing a sign on the closet door, dresser or bedside table that has the word describing the article and a picture of it may be all that is needed. A large sign on the closet door with the words and pictures indicating shirts, pants, shoes and a sign showing a pipe, hair brush, etc. on the bedside door compensates for my memory loss. Before using any signs, it is again important to assess the client's ability to read and understand either the pictures or the words.

Locator signs on washroom doors, whether the door is accessed from within the client's room or from the hall, are necessary. The sign must be bright, contrasting against the color of the door, large, with the word "washroom" and a picture of a toilet. Even though the washroom may be attached to a client's room, the person will probably not find it if the door is closed. She will wander into the hallway, looking for the toilet. The delay may result in the client being incontinent. This demonstrates that it is important to leave nothing to memory. If the client cannot see it, he probably cannot find it.

Mirrors

Most of us have an "internal picture" of ourselves. This can be demonstrated simply enough. How many times has someone taken a snapshot of you and you exclaimed - "That's not me. I don't look like that." That snapshot is in conflict with your own internal picture, how you believe you look.

At this moment what can you see of yourself?

Your hands, the rest of your body, but you cannot see your face. The only time you have an opportunity to see your face is when you look in the mirror.

The same is true with a mentally impaired client. If a mentally impaired client sees himself as 42 years old, but in actual fact he is 85, there is nothing to contradict that perception.

Like everything else discussed, mirrors:

- are of value for some mentally impaired
- create agitation in others
- elicit peculiar responses in still others
- are completely oblivious to the remainder

A mirror can cause agitated behavior in some mentally impaired. If a mentally impaired client has the ability to know that he is looking at his reflection in a mirror, he will experience considerable difficulty. Due to his memory loss, he sees himself in his mind as 42 years old, but in actual fact he is 84. Looking at his reflection he will experience a state called Reality Shock.

This is a situation where the person is suddenly confronted with something that contradicts his beliefs. When this client sees his reflection in the mirror and he knows it is him, the contradiction creates intense and immediate confusion. His anxiety level then increases to a panic state, he becomes agitated and may break the mirror. For this individual, a mirror must not be in his room.

Other mentally impaired clients do not have the cognitive ability to know that they are seeing their own reflection when they look in a mirror. The mirror in this situation then initiates a very different behavioral response. This client will talk to their reflection, believing it is someone else.

The stimulus for this person is too obscure. It causes him to misinterpret what he sees. In fact, the mirror may result in an 82 year old client telling you that he just saw his father, when in actual fact, he was looking at himself. There is no question that the location of a mirror for this client is of significant importance. If a mirror is located in this client's room where he can see it while lying in bed, then he may be very restless at night and unable to sleep. It would be rude to sleep when you have a visitor, or frightening if you believed there was someone else in the room that you did not know.

The location of a mirror must be considered carefully. In one facility a full length mirror was at the end of the hall. It was interesting to watch certain mentally impaired clients walk down the hall. As they caught sight of themselves in the mirror, they stepped to the other side of the hall, and then moved back again. Obviously they were trying to get out of the way of the person coming towards them (seeing their own reflection in the mirror). A mirror in this location can contribute to some clients falling or becoming aggressive, getting angry when they cannot get out of the way of the other person.

The majority of dementia clients (level two) cannot use a mirror and will often misinterpret the image seen in the mirror. Mirrors need to be removed or camouflaged to decrease the confusion that can be created.

Glass covering pictures or paintings on the hallway walls may cause a similar response as mirrors. Non-glare glass should be used. If not, the picture will be lost and the mentally impaired client will talk to his reflection.

Hooking Old Memory

If the lounge looks like a waiting room, the client will wait for only so long and if nothing happens she will leave. If the dining room is just a large room with a number of tables in it, then a dementia client will have a problem sitting there to eat. The dining room must look like a dining room and the lounge look like a living room. A dementia client does not need to be told what to do when he sees a sofa, he sits. He does not need to be told where to eat when he sees the proper table.

If old memory is hooked, the chances are great that a mentally impaired client may respond appropriately to what he/she is seeing. Furniture is now available that is attractive and home-like in appearance, but easy to maintain and treated against incontinence. Using end tables, table lamps and floor lamps adds the needed touch. To eliminate the concern that lamps may be knocked over, they only need to be secured to the table from the bottom (similar to what is done in motel rooms), and floor lamps secured to the floor. The more the room can look normal, the more the behavior it elicits will be normal.

Plants, pictures, books, book shelves are all essential in any living environment. Pictures on the walls need only be secured by screwing them to the wall so that they are not easily knocked down or used as weapons.

Multiple Lounges/Alternate Dining Rooms

An appropriate living environment for the mentally impaired must be one that limits the amount of stimuli that can be encountered. One large lounge with thirty or more clients is too much activity for most who are mentally impaired, especially if that lounge is also where the radio and TV are located.

It is important to separate those clients who can easily agitate others from those who are sensitive to such stimuli. Multiple small lounges allow clients to be placed in a room that best suits them. Usually three smaller lounges are best - a TV room, a music room and a quiet room. This provides the needed flexibility in locating clients based on their functioning ability and sensitivity to stimuli.

For some clients, having a comfortable chair and a radio in their room may be a viable option. This allows the opportunity to provide certain clients periods alone in a quiet environment.

The dining room must be versatile. Clients who are able to feed themselves, but are easily distracted, require little to take their attention from their meal. A small dining room is needed for those who can be disruptive to allow higher functioning mentally impaired clients to concentrate on their meal without being distracted.

Parks

An outside enclosed park is an asset to any unit. A park enclosed by a chain linked fence is not sufficient. Certain wanderers may leave an enclosed area, not from the desire to leave the building or property, but only from being attracted to what they see on the other side of the fence - children playing, or a garden that needs tending in the next yard. A chain linked fence allows the mentally impaired client to see what is on the other side, resulting in some scaling over the top and leaving the courtyard.

The best enclosure is one that appears as a solid wall to the mentally impaired, such as hedging in front of a louvered wooden fence (see book case design in chapter on Wandering). Even though one can see through the fence at a certain angle, to the mentally impaired the wall appears solid, decreasing the tendency to go over the wall to the next yard.

The walking path in the park needs to be a winding walkway that starts and ends at the door to the unit. When the client walks the path, he is virtually led away and back to the unit - he will wander the unit, go out the door, wander in the park and return to wander the unit, a never ending loop.

The ideal park is one that is landscaped with bushes, a gazebo and benches strategically placed so the wanderer has resting points. These resting stations need something to attract him to stop, such as raised gardens or flower beds which bring the plants into view and allow the client to till the soil or touch the flowers or pick them without stooping. Bird feeders add a nice touch.

Unfortunately some very attractive and functional enclosed courtyards for the mentally impaired are rarely used. On a majority of units, the mentally impaired are often told directly or indirectly (by security devices), not to go out any doors. Yet they are being told (during nice weather only) to go out the door that leads to the courtyard. The clients do not have the cognitive ability to function under such confusing and contradictory instructions.

The only way the mentally impaired will utilize a courtyard is if they are drawn out. Placing an automatic opening patio door in the wandering path is one answer. As the wanderer crosses the sensor to the patio door, it opens. The person will then be attracted through it (looking for something familiar) and will walk the leading pathway (starts and ends at the patio door) through the courtyard. On returning to the door, the sensor will be activated again, the patio door will open and the person will enter the unit. The process is repeated continually. In this way the unit has created an effective wandering loop. By the way, if the weather is poor, just flip the switch to the patio door, shutting off the sensor. The client will walk up to the door, nothing happens, he will then move down the hall.

P.A. System

> You are a mentally impaired client
> Living in a long term care facility./
> You are sitting alone in the lounge./
> Suddenly there is a voice from nowhere./
>
> What is your response?

As soon as the P.A. speaker sounds off with a message, some mentally impaired clients begin talking aloud. It takes a great deal of cognitive ability to know the voice is coming from a speaker, connected by wire to the front office.

Even cognitively well clients in most facilities do not relate to random P.A. announcements. How often do activity staff go to the unit to get clients for an activity even though the announcement was just made? By the time a cognitively well client is aware that the message concerns her and she is attentive, the message is over. This even happens to staff. How often has someone come to you and said, "That page was for you, didn't you hear it?"

Unnecessary noise must be eliminated. The most appropriate use of the P.A. is to establish a specific time each morning for all client announcements. Having announcements each morning between 0900 and 0910 hours encourages the cognitively well clients to be more attentive, rather than having to listen to the barrage of random messages bombarding them each day. The goal is to eliminate the use of the P.A. systems. Supplying key personnel with a beeper (maintenance staff, administrator, director of nursing), and restricting the P.A. to emergency calls only, will make the environment a much quieter and more comfortable setting for all concerned.

Television

Many mentally impaired clients are incapable of watching TV. Imagine sitting in a chair when you suddenly hear from behind you "Don't turn around. If you turn around there is nothing I can do but shoot you in the back." That is what can be heard from a TV. Imagine how a dementia client would respond not knowing the source of the statement.

A TV program moves too fast from one scene to another - at one moment the client is watching a soap commercial and the next she sees a car blow up. Those mentally impaired who do watch TV, probably do so from old behavior and old memory. Ask a male, mentally impaired client watching a hockey game who is playing and what is the score, and he will be unable to tell you. If he is able to sit for extended periods in front of the TV during a hockey game, it is likely old behavior for him. He has watched hockey games all of his life and the behavior is familiar to him. Similarly, another client may be watching a soap opera and know nothing of what is happening or who is involved. Again, it may only be old behavior. On the other hand, playing nature scenes with soft music utilizing a VCR or DVD player becomes excellent programming for the dementia client.

Unfortunately, turning on the TV becomes an immediate habit of some caregivers. As soon as they walk into the lounge, the TV is switched on and left on all day. The care team must be consciously aware to decrease the amount of stimuli on the unit at all times. There are certain noises and disruptions that cannot be avoided , however those that can be controlled must be eliminated.

If the TV in the lounge is located on the floor, it will attract the wandering clients. The wanderer is often drawn to the greatest stimuli. Frequently this client walks to the TV, stands in front of it, strokes it, turns the dials, etc. This sets the stage for a potential aggressive outburst from those watching the program (on a mixed unit which includes cognitively well clients). To solve the problem, the TV need only be attached to the wall at above eye level and tilted slightly forward. This keeps the TV out of view from the wanderer, making him less likely to disrupt others watching it.

Placing the TV at such a height then becomes an inconvenience for those who want to choose the channel and control the volume. What is needed is a remote controlled TV, where the remote control is secured to a table top where the cognitively well clients sit. This allows them to be independent while watching TV, and the remote control is too small for the mentally impaired to be attracted to it.

If the volume of the TV needs to be loud for it to be heard, it creates even more noise. External speakers can be installed to address the volume issue. These speakers can be located at the back of the lounge allowing those clients who are watching a program to hear it and still keep the volume low. If a cognitively well client has a hearing problem and needs the volume higher than anyone else, attaching volume controlled earphones to the speakers allows this client to hear the program without disturbing others.

Music

The tempo, the accentuated down beat and the periodic unintelligible lyrics of modern music has the potential of agitating the mentally impaired. Soothing conventional music has the opposite effect, and is more relaxing. In fact, the right music is playing when many young staff complain that they do not like the radio station.

As with everything else we have discussed, music to some mentally impaired clients is noise to others. Constant music piped in over the P.A. system can create sensory overload for the mentally impaired or anyone else for that matter.

Why is it that during a meeting in the board room, staff or managers want the P.A. turned off?

To demonstrate the impact of such constant stimuli, leave the piped in music on during your next meeting and see how difficult it is for all to concentrate on what is being said. This exercise usually results in the music being turned off in the halls. The goal in the environment of the mentally impaired is to decrease stimuli.

Fire Drills

Fire drills can create the most havoc with the mentally impaired. Of course there is no value to warn staff in advance of a pending fire drill, but it is necessary to be prepared for its effects. The anxiety level of the mentally impaired is increased dramatically during the drill. The ability of any client to immediately respond to any further stress afterwards is severely restricted. Trying to bath a mentally impaired client who has just gone through a fire drill that he does not understand is impossible. Trying to run a scheduled activity program with a group of mentally impaired clients just after a fire drill is useless. The mentally impaired must be allowed to settle before the routine of the unit is resumed. Whoever is pulling the fire alarm must know that for at least one to two hours afterwards, activities involving mentally impaired clients are canceled or postponed until "things return to normal."

Staff Identification

Staff name tags are necessary and commonly used. Name tags that are small, with small printing, containing too much information or have a shiny surface (brass or gold), are of little value. Name tags need to be large with the staff member's first name only. There is no need for the department to be identified on the name tag, those words have little meaning to many of the mentally impaired. Color coding name tags to identify departments may have a better impact - red for housekeeping, blue for nursing, etc.

Working with the mentally impaired requires an investment of energy into new and innovative techniques and approaches. We are forging a new philosophy in what we do and how we do it. Our success can be measured by the response of the clients within our care.

Chapter Fifteen

Specialization

Long term care (as well as acute care and community based programs) has experienced major transitions over the years. Initially, the client population within long term care facilities averaged 74 years of age and represented individuals requiring minimal supports. The care practices during that time were more of a residential model. The picture began to change in the late 1980's when the client population averaged 85 to 87 years in age and the clientele became physically frail and more incapacitated. This required a shift to a clinical model of care. The new transition of today involves the mentally impaired elderly. Most long term care facilities have a client population where 70% are mentally impaired, with many presenting an array of behaviors, some demonstrating high risk behaviors. The required model today is behavioral care.

These changing demands require facilities to develop the skills and resources to manage the complex needs of mentally impaired clients. When the expertise of the care team does not at least match the needs of the client being served then the outcomes can be quite negative. The following are some examples of what has occurred in recent years:

- A dementia client drinking a caustic solution from an unattended and unsecured housekeeping cart, seriously damaging her esophagus, resulting in the need for a tracheotomy and G tube.
- A dementia client wandering out of a facility during the winter because of an improper mag lock device used to

secure the exit doors, a problem known by all within that facility, the lady died of exposure.

- A newly admitted dementia client beating two other dementia clients to death with the foot rest of a wheelchair, as well as seriously injuring two other clients and two caregivers.
- A dementia client wandering off a hospital medical unit, despite an intense search the individual was not located until a month later wedged behind a boiler, dead.

These are not isolated incidences. Nor do these incidents reflect facilities that are notorious for providing poor care. On the contrary, these are good facilities who were not equipped to manage the mentally impaired elderly with challenging behaviors.

These cases traumatized everyone involved. Those within the facilities questioned how it could happen. When the situation was assessed, the question was more "How did it not happen before this incident?"

The challenges of caring effectively for the mentally impaired elderly will not be one that lessens, but only intensifies. All sectors - long term care, acute care and community care, have more than one client presenting high risk behaviors.

The following section identifies three areas for consideration in creating a culture that emphasizes behavioral care. It is important to determine how the outcomes outlined in these initiatives can be achieved within your setting. The areas include:

- Behavioral Care Practices Manual
- Performance Audits
- Modular Care

Behavioral Care Practices Manual

The need for a Behavioral Care Practices Manual is based on two important issues:

1) Each caregiver has different experiences, abilities and skills.
2) It is necessary to differentiate the practices that apply to the mentally impaired from those that apply to the cognitively well

1) Caregiver Performance

Caregivers present different performance abilities. The graph represents the levels of expertise in behavior care and behavior management. The solid dashes represent the different performance levels of caregivers within a care team.

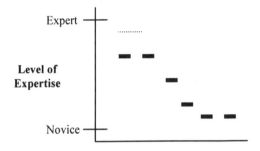

Some caregivers are highly skilled in working with the mentally impaired (represented by the solid dashes at the top of the scale). Their ability to determine needs, read behavioral cues and respond with appropriate supportive measures allows them a degree of success with or without the use of formal tools or direction from others. Other caregivers do not have the same experience, training, or innate ability to perform at that level or achieve the same results (represented by the solid dashes at the bottom of the scale). This disparity in performance levels can often create significant conflict, disagreements and inconsistencies within the care team.

If no efforts are made to balance performance levels, then introducing complicated and sophisticated behavior management tools to address the needs of high risk behaviors (represented by the dotted line at the top of the graph) are destined for failure. To introduce such tools to a care team without an established culture of effective behavioral care practices will only distance care performance and intensify the conflicts. Those who are highly skilled become excited about the introduction of these tools, and are able to use them to their full potential. However, those with less ability (those at the bottom of the graph) do not achieve the same results. On the contrary, these caregivers cannot understand the value of such complex tools, how to interpret them or how to use the information they generate. The tool becomes just another task to perform, a waste of time.

A Behavioral Care Practices Manual is a guidebook that allows less skilled caregivers to replicate the abilities of those who are intuitively skilled. Once there is commonality in performance then more complex behavior management tools can be introduced to successfully address the needs of high risk behaviors.

2) Defining Behavioral Care

Without a Behavior Management Practices Manual each caregiver is left to determine how clinical practices must be adapted to the different clients they encounter. For example, in many organizations the same admission practices are generally applied to all clients regardless of the person's functioning ability. As demonstrated earlier, admission practices involving the mentally impaired are very defined and highly specific. When the differences in admission, assessment, programming, analysis, etc. are not defined, then it is left to the proficiency level and understanding of the individual caregiver to determine what should or should not be done. Given the graph above, each caregiver will have a different interpretation of what is needed and create different outcomes.

The purpose of a Behavioral Care Practices Manual is to provide all caregivers with the direction on what is to be done for this clientele. This ensures consistency in performance and results. The major components of a Practices Manual are as follows:

> *Foundations for Care*
> *Admission*
> *Assessment*
> *Analysis*

Programming
Environment
Family/Caregiver Support
Outcome Measurements
Care Analysis Reference Section

The benefits gained from a Behavioral Care Practices Manual are many:

- Demonstrates the differences in care practices with dementia clients (especially those with challenging behaviors) from those used with cognitively well clients.
- Provides a guidebook for all team members on the tools used, when they are to be implemented, the rationale for their use and how they are to be used.
- Enhances consistency in performance.
- Provides an excellent orientation and training manual for new employees.
- Ideal reference to identify for family the specialization of care for their family member.
- Creates a competitive edge by defining the care differences found in this facility compared to others.
- Provides a baseline from which to hold caregivers accountable.
- Excellent care practices reference document in the event of legal action taken due to the actions of a high risk dementia client.
- Defines the ability to admit and manage high risk clients.
- Provides transfer locations (i.e. acute care) detailed direction on existing practices, allowing proper interpretation and use of accompanying information on client being transferred.
- Assists behavioral consults to know existing practices and information sources.
- Establishes outcome measurement criteria to determine effectiveness of care.

Supportive Therapy provides the content for a Behavioral Care Practices Manual (presented throughout this text and in the text "Preventing Alzheimer's Aggression: Supportive Therapy in Action"). However, Supportive Therapy is not a "take it or leave it" modality. It has been developed to provide flexibility in its implementation:

- It can be replicated in its entirety.
- Any portion can be used by a facility to enhance existing practices.
- It can be used as a comparison benchmark to evaluate existing facility practices.

To be effective organizations need to develop a site specific Behavioral Care Practices Manual. This requires identifying what is in place that is working; what is outdated and needs to be replaced or enhanced; what is missing. The following is a detailed content list of the components of a Behavioral Care Practices Manual. Define next to each item what exists in your organization.

Behavioral Care Practices Manual

Foundations for Care
- the philosophy of care for:
  o the dementia client
  o dementia clients demonstrating challenging behaviors
  o use of physical restraints
  o use of psychotropic medication or chemical restraints
- the principals from which care is defined
- the objectives to be achieved
- expectations of the care team
- expectations regarding the consistency of care
- who is responsible for assessing challenging behaviors and who is involved in determining the direction for care
- expectations when high risk behaviors are encountered

Admission
- family information package
- admission questionnaire
- pre admission conference
- admission conference
- post admission conference
- day of admission
- week after admission
- month after admission
- staff assignment to a new admission
- family support pre and post admission
- belongings and room layout

Assessment
- medical
- medication
- functional
- activities of daily living (ADL)
- interview
- programming
- medication
- behavioral
- environmental

Analysis
- analysis mechanism when a behavior occurs
- method to differentiate causes of a behavior
- mechanism of analyzing behavior during a care conference
- how knowledge of those who know the client (secrets) is tapped
- how information is communicated to the care team
- how supportive measures are identified
- how outcomes or results from supportive measures are determined

- how shift report is conducted for those with challenging behaviors

Programming
- list of programming options available (large group, small group and one-to-one)
- who conducts programming
- tool to monitor and evaluate a client's involvement in programming (during and after)
- mechanism for non-recreation staff to know exactly what programs a client is involved in, how they are set-up, what to expect from the client, how and when they should be used, etc.
- assessment mechanism to determine the most appropriate program and when needed
- method to evaluate programming options
- how consults (physiotherapist, OT) are used to assist with challenging behaviors

Environment
- environmental adaptations to accommodate dementia clients in general, as well as specific adaptations for those with challenging behaviors (i.e. wandering, aggression, mimicking, etc.)
- cueing techniques, why they are used, how they are assessed
- methods to control stimuli (traffic flow, noise, lighting, etc.)
- safety factors addressed (exit doors, weapons, etc.)

Family/Caregiver Support
- how family are helped to understand dementia and behavior
- how family concerns are approached and resolved
- how information is communicated to family
- how family are helped to understand other clients they may contact during their visit
- how family are helped to manage the behaviors of other clients they may contact

- resources available to assist family (i.e. Alzheimer's Society, family and counseling services)
- how caregivers are supported when they encounter behaviors they have difficulty managing (i.e. sexual, violent)
- client advocacy program
- orientation package that assists new staff to understand the dementia client and their behaviors
- how new staff, family and volunteers are mentored or supported to deal with hard to manage clients
- number of volunteers available, number who work directly with dementia clients, number who work with dementia clients with challenging behaviors
- how volunteers are trained and the role they play in programming
- specialized resources available (i.e. psychogeriatrician, behavioral team, etc.) and how they are used

Performance Audits
- method to communicate concerns about high risk clients
- who those concerns are communicated to and expected actions taken
- involvement of the care team in determining the actions to be taken and evaluating the results
- how psychotropic medication is monitored and evaluated
- how the environment is evaluated to determine appropriateness for changing client needs and safety issues
- how the care team is assessed to determine consistency in care
- how programs are monitored and evaluated to determine appropriateness for existing client population

Behavioral Reference Section
(identified as Care Analysis Reference Section)
- listing of all behaviors (aggression, sexually expressive, wandering, rummaging/hoarding, ingestion of foreign objectives, repetitive, etc.)

- reference list of potential causes for each behavior
- recommended supportive measures for each cause

If there was difficulty in detailing and completing this list then you may have identified what may be creating the frustrations and inconsistencies in managing challenging behaviors within your setting.

Present this list to a group of staff and management representatives from all departments within your organization. Collectively define what exists and what is needed. This will assist in developing the culture to meet the special needs of the mentally impaired with challenging behaviors.

Performance Audits

Performance Audits are tools used to identify a care team's level of expertise and provide direction on areas requiring attention or development. The following are examples of Performance Audits covering a variety of areas:

Psychotropic Audit

A Psychotropic Audit defines the use of psychotropic medication (both regularly dispensed and PRN) to manage behaviors. The following is required for a Psychotropic Audit:

- number of clients on a unit
- number of clients on a unit who are mentally impaired
- number of mentally impaired clients not receiving psychotropic medication (to determine actual number of medications per client)
- number of regularly dispensed psychotropic medications
- number of PRN psychotropic medications
- number of PRN psychotropic medications dispensed:
  - o more than once per day over the past month

- o less than five times per week over the past month
- o not used in the past month
- number of psychotropic medications used for HS purposes only
- number of clients on more than one regularly dispensed or PRN psychotropic medication

The results identify the dependency on psychotropic medication to manage behaviors and the need for alternate strategies; provide a base line from which to measure the benefits gained from implementation of specific behavioral care practices; and establishes needed outcome targets to enhance performance. Interpretation of the results will reveal the following:

- Any category where there is a high use of psychotropic medication requires more detailed investigation into the specific clients involved, evaluating the care practices used with these clients and examination of alternate approaches.

- Comparing audit results from previous months will indicate the impact of newly implemented behavioral care practices.

- The audit defines performance targets for psychotropic medication use. Once the baseline of existing use is identified, the care team is to achieve a 10% decrease in the use of psychotropic medication by the next audit. This requires the care team to initiate new practices or further enhance existing ones. Once the new baseline is achieved, the care team is to decrease psychotropic medication use again by 10%. This is repeated until it is felt that the use of psychotropic medication is at its minimum therapeutic level (supporting a minimal restraint policy).

Practices Audit
A Practices Audit is used to determine if revisions are needed to existing procedures or policies. A form of a Shadow Assessment is

used to evaluate existing practices. This involves shadowing or observing a dementia client with challenging behaviors for an extended period to identify:

- routines and procedures the client is exposed to.
- the client's response or potential negative impact the client may experience.
- possible alternative actions that should be taken.

The findings of the Practices Audit are then analyzed to determine which routines and procedures require revision to meet the specific needs of those with dementia, especially those demonstrating challenging behaviors.

Care Plan Audit

A Care Plan Audit determines the consistency of knowledge and practices of the care team. A Care Plan Audit involves identifying five caregivers from different departments who are in contact with a specific client demonstrating challenging behaviors. Each caregiver is interviewed separately about the client, examples of the questions asked include:

How do you approach this client?
How do you get him to the dining room?
How do you get him to sit down?
How do you get him to eat his meal?
What do you do when he becomes upset or disruptive?

If answers to these questions are not consistent, then a review of existing practices is in order.

Environmental Audits

1) Global Environmental Audit - yearly audit involving representatives from all departments and all levels of staff and managers to identify concerns regarding safety issues; lighting/heating problems; noise level and wandering path

concerns; furniture, equipment and programming needs; overcrowding and underutilization of areas or rooms.

2) Safety Audit - consists of a formally documented environmental safety audit conducted quarterly by a senior manager to identify possible safety issues, i.e. hallway clutter, unlocked non-client room doors, access to poisonous/caustic solutions, unsafe equipment, potential weapons, unattended cleaning equipment and solutions, etc.

Program Involvement

A Program Audit determines which clients receive recreational programs and areas where new programming is required (note a Programming Audit is not necessary if a Programming Map is in place). A Programming Audit involves:

- Listing all mentally impaired clients on a unit.
- Identifying the number of clients usually involved in a large group activity (i.e. 10 or more).
- Eliminating all large group programs (i.e. programs involving 10 or more), recreation staff are to identify the number of dementia clients involved in:
  - 7 or more activities per week
  - 3 to 7 activities per week
  - less than 3 activities per week
- individuals attending less than 3 activities per week are identified.
- recreation staff are to identify which new programs will be developed for these individuals to increase their opportunity for participation.

Behavioral Audit

It is important that the management team monitor possible safety issues and potential liability risks. A quarterly Behavioral Audit provides the management team with the following information:

- the number of clients with high risk behaviors and steps taken to decrease the risk factor
- the number of psychotropic medications and restraints used, steps taken to decrease their use
- unit safety issues or concerns identified by the care team and steps taken to resolve them
- family complaints regarding clients demonstrating high risk behaviors and how they are resolved
- caregiver and client injuries resulting from high risk behaviors, steps taken to prevent the re-occurrence of these injuries

Information provided from a behavioral audit is necessary to evaluate existing practices and develop a strategic plan to enhance performance.

Modular Care

It is important regardless of where you work to read these next pages. The end of this section provides a way to determine how the needs of level two dementia clients are met whether they live in a specialized environment or an integrated setting.

There has been considerable controversy whether the mentally impaired client should be on the same unit as the cognitively well/physically disabled client, or located on a separate unit with like clients. If the question is one of segregation, without the provision of appropriate supports, then the answer is a simple one - no! To segregate is to take from view or remove from sight. If that is the intention of such a unit then it should never be considered. Without a well-structured plan of action and clear-cut guidelines, such a unit can easily become a "dumping ground" - a location where any "difficult" client is placed to prevent him from disturbing others. Unfortunately, some facilities have such a unit - very little programming, no admission or discharge criteria, untrained staff and so on. These are the ones that give autonomous units for the mentally impaired an undeserved reputation.

Most facilities employ a form of autonomy to some degree or another even though they may not have a separate unit for the mentally impaired. It is common to find many clients located on specific units or floors based on need and functioning. Level two mentally impaired clients who have a tendency to wander are often placed on the second floor to make it more difficult for them to leave the building. Units are often divided where heavy physical care clients are located on one floor or unit, ambulatory/well clients on another and so on.

By the way, if the facility does not take the steps to place the mentally impaired clients in one area or on one unit, then the cognitively well clients will employ some form of separation on their own. When a unit is totally integrated, many cognitively well clients are found sitting in the lounge in the front lobby, in an activity room or in their room in order to stay away from the behaviors encountered in the more common areas.

A unit for the mentally impaired is selective in who it serves. The level one mentally impaired, the individual who is aware there is a problem and is still able to function with minimal supports, does not require such a specialized setting. Likewise, level three of functioning, or those who are severely impaired both mentally and physically, do not require such a unit. A unit for the mentally impaired is specifically intended for the mentally impaired at level two of functioning - those who are physically well, experiencing a considerable degree of impairment, and require specific and intense supports.

One of the criticisms of developing specialized units is that it contradicts the concept of "aging in place." However, the present belief that aging in place means the person must remain in the same room is too restrictive. There are two problems with this concept.

1) Few facilities have the resources to maintain such a restrictive mode of operation. Attempting to stretch resources and staffing to meet the variety of needs of all clients scattered throughout the

building, usually results in an inefficient utilization of resources and ineffective care. In reality, long term care represents multiple specialties:

- cognitively well clients requiring a minimal to moderate level of care
- individuals requiring a high level of physical care
- those who are confused and disoriented
- the confused and disoriented who demonstrate challenging behaviors

Caregivers cannot be everything to everyone and still achieve maximum efficiency and effectiveness.

2) Likewise, the specific needs of clients cannot be adequately met in an integrated environment. In an integrated environment, there is always a struggle over who receives the caregivers' time and attention.
   - Those who are the most frail can receive the least amount of care because the more independent cognitively well are able to speak up and dominate the caregiver's time.
   - If that is not the case then the attentions of those who are the most frail become the caregiver's priority, resulting in the more independent client becoming dissatisfied with the care and service they receive, causing them to complain to family and potentially tainting the reputation of the facility.
   - Similarly, the confused that demonstrate challenging behaviors can take a great deal of caregiver's time, leaving those who are mildly confused overlooked.
   - If the latter does not occur, then those with the most challenging behaviors must be controlled, resulting in their being heavily medicated and restrained, unnecessarily increasing the workload and negatively impacting on the reputation of the facility.

This tug-of-war for resources can create an inefficiency where all may be negatively affected.

"Aging in place" must apply to the building, not to the bed where the person was first admitted. The concept of developing specialized units is called Modular Care. Although transferring from unit to unit is a concern, it is kept to a minimum and is as much a part of programming as any other aspect of care. A Behavioral Care Practices manual ensures that the depth of knowledge and understanding about each client is transferred with them and care is replicated with minimal distress and maximum benefit.

Modular Care provides a number of benefits to the organization, it's staff, managers and clients. These include:

- the opportunity for staff to:
    - specialize in an area best suited to their ability and interest, enhancing job performance
    - receive comprehensive training in a specific specialty area, enhancing efficiency and performance
    - be a member of a specialized unit, increasing ownership and willingness to take on responsibilities
    - achieve optimum job satisfaction, positively impacting on retention and recruitment
- the opportunity for clients to:
    - benefit from best practices related to a specialized care setting, optimizing client functioning ability and quality of life
    - receive the most appropriate support based on their personal functioning ability, creating a more positive living environment
    - receive individualized care, enhancing client and family satisfaction
- the opportunity for the organization to:
    - create four specialized units within one building, providing a more efficient operation

- re-structure into smaller autonomous, self contained units, which can optimize use of resources, enhance efficiency and improve cost effectiveness
- increase its profile within the community and the industry at large, enhancing marketability, increasing optimum occupancy rates, providing greater financial return and becoming a stronger employment draw

It is important to emphasize that no model can be 100% effective in achieving its desired end. Although specific units are based on functioning ability, the reality is simple - when beds are available, they must be filled. However, with this model internal transfers become the priority. When a bed becomes available, existing clients are transferred within the building to the location where they will receive maximum benefit. Once internal transfers are complete, then admissions from the community are sought to best fit the available bed.

Overview of Modular Care

Modular Care involves dividing a facility into four specialized areas. Of course the size of the facility and the number of dementia clients within the facility will dictate the extent and feasibility of such an initiative. Newly built long term care facilities designed in a pod construction, housing 24 to 25 clients per pod, are the most suitable to develop specialized environments. An overview of the four specialty areas is as follows;

Cognitively Well Unit (CCWU),
Physical Care Unit (PCU).
Dementia Unit (DU),
Dementia Special Needs Unit (DSNU),

Cognitively Well Unit (CWU)
This unit houses cognitively well clients who require care but still demonstrate a degree of independence and control over their surroundings. The intention of this unit is to develop a living environment that has a shared governance with the clients in defining unit routines, expectations, etc. The focus of this unit is customer service. Programming, environmental décor, staff training, assessment tools, etc. allow the care team to match the care practices and routines with the desires of the client and his family.

Physical Care Unit (PCU)
This specialized unit houses both cognitively well and mentally impaired clients who require complex physical care. The resources available to this unit are greater than the Cognitively Well and Dementia Units. The care team would be skilled in developing care strategies specific to the needs of this population and considered specialists in Palliative Care.

Dementia Special Needs Unit (DSNU)
The profile of a Dementia Special Needs Unit (DSNU) would be:
- Housing ambulatory dementia clients only.
- The care team is skilled in behavior management techniques to address high risk behaviors.
- Specialized behavior management assessment, care and programming tools are available.
- Higher caregiver/client ratio.
- Dementia specific environmental designs and supports for high risk behaviors.
- Defined and rigidly maintained admission and discharge criteria.
- Consistently assigned recreation staff skilled in programming development with challenging behaviors.
- Access to professional consults.
- Minimal use of chemical and physical restraints.
- Primary objective is to stabilize and discharge.

- Considered a closed unit, access can be restricted if deemed inappropriate for the circumstances occurring on the unit at the time.
- Ideal bed capacity: 14 to a maximum of 24.

An admission/discharge criteria must be developed for a DSNU, without a defined criteria the unit has the potential to admit inappropriate clients and retain those who can no longer benefit from living on the unit. Standard admission criteria, other than impairment in mental ability, is based on the client's response to any other living environment including:

- Behavior – behaviors that are difficult to manage (including aggression, wandering, elopement, sexual expressive, repetitive, etc.) requiring a care team skilled in behavior management.
- Restrained or Highly Medicated – individuals who risk being restrained or heavily medicated to control their behaviors if they lived on any other unit.
- Require a Controlled Environment – individuals who are susceptible to noise, stimuli, etc., resulting in challenging behaviors or consistent, visible signs of distress.
- Flexible Care Routine – individuals who require *continuous* flexibility in their care routine that cannot be achieved elsewhere within the facility and if not achieved will result in challenging behaviors or consistent, visible signs of distress.
- Ridiculed – individuals who are or can be ridiculed by cognitively well or high functioning dementia clients resulting in challenging behaviors or consistent, visible signs of distress.
- Minimum Programming Involvement – individuals who would benefit from specialized programming offered by a Dementia Special Needs Unit, which is not offered elsewhere in the facility.

The admission notes must record why the individual was admitted to the DSNU (as defined by the admission criteria) and what the individual will gain from this unit that cannot be found elsewhere in the building, excluding a secured door.

Furthermore, the physical environmental of a DSNU must contribute to behavior management practices. Environmental components include:

- a secured unit to provide safe wandering and eliminate the elopement risk.
- a wandering path that leads clients to programming areas and away from high sensitive areas.
- access to an exterior courtyard with a defined circular wandering path.
- the ability to separate highly volatile clients from those who are disruptive.
- minimal exposure to disruptive stimuli (noise, lighting, glare) and congestion.
- homelike, to enhance client functioning ability and way finding.
- multiple location anchors to enhance way finding and orientation.
- specialized safety features specific to those with dementia and high risk behaviors.

The philosophy of a Dementia Special Needs Unit is to discharge the client as soon as possible. This requires the unit to be highly skilled in assessment and programming practices to establish the most appropriate approach and supportive strategies to resolve challenging behaviors and enhance functioning ability. The discharge criteria is identified on admission (defined in the admission notes, as outlined above). Once the original objectives for admission are achieved, the original need or behavior has been stabilized or no longer exists, and no new further challenges are encountered, then the client can be transferred to a Dementia Unit or Sister Unit.

Dementia Unit (DU)

A Dementia Unit is a sister unit to a DSNU. The success of any DSNU is based on an available sister dementia care unit. Without a sister dementia unit:

- clients are often held on a DSNU too long
- a "revolving door syndrome" results where clients who are transferred are returned to the unit because care practices are not maintained
- inappropriate admissions occur because there is no alternative available

A sister unit parallels the behavioral care assessment tools and programming of a DSNU, but does not have the same caregiver/client ratio and only houses dementia clients when their behavior is stabilized. The profile of a Dementia Unit is:

- houses:
  - higher functioning dementia clients who require support and care, who do not demonstrate challenging behaviors on a regular basis and who do not require a specialized environment
  - non-ambulatory dementia clients who do not require high levels of physical care
  - the primary unit from which transfers to the DSNU are received when the behavior of those clients stabilizes, resulting in no further need for a secured or controlled environment, or ongoing behavior management interventions
- programming, environment, staff training, assessment tools, etc., would be at a behavioral care level identical with the DSNU
- an open unit (no access restriction)
- the resources on this unit would be less than those on a DSNU

Modular Care Exercise

Implementation of Modular Care is a major cultural shift for some facilities. The decision cannot be made simply on the projected challenges such a shift may create or the desire to hold onto the existing philosophy of care. Those facilities who have an integrated environment as well as those with autonomous units must continually identify the strengths and challenges each presents. Examining the feasibility of Modular Care provides a facility the opportunity to evaluate their existing model of care. An excellent quality improvement and strategic planning exercise involves:

- identifying the pros and cons of an integrated environment
- identifying the pros and cons of Modular Care
- then examining how the cons of each method can be resolved

Maintaining the status quo without resolving the limitations the present system creates would decrease the effectiveness of any efforts taken. Ruling out Modular Care without an analysis of whether the concerns regarding changing to that method can be address would be shortsighted. The completion of this exercise will define what needs to be done should the status quo be maintained or what is required should Modular Care be implemented.

Chapter Sixteen

Outcome Measurement

Quality of Life Indicators for
The Mentally Impaired Elderly

The following is an overview of many of the components required to successfully provide behavioral care to the mentally impaired elderly in long term care facilities. To determine the strengths and weaknesses of your facility in this area, check the appropriate number next to each statement. The numbers represent the following code:

1) In place and working.
2) In place, but needs further development or is not consistent.
3) Non-existent.

1 2 3   PHILOSOPHY

___ ___ ___   1) The philosophy of care establishes that these clients are to be treated as "normal" functioning adults without expectations of "normal" behavior. This is communicated, understood and practiced by all staff.

___ ___ ___   2) Staff know that all behavior has meaning. Periodic aggressive or resistive outbursts are acceptable behavior, understanding that for some this is the only means to communicate their frustration. Behavioral responses are regularly assessed to determine how to best support this individual.

___ ___ ___ 3) Staff are taught to maintain physical contact (touching, holding, hugging, etc.) beyond times of performing basic care tasks.

___ ___ ___ 4) Staff have accepted that certain behaviors (i.e. wandering, repetitive behaviors, etc.) do not require intervention unless they create negative consequences.

___ ___ ___ 5) The cognitively well clients in contact with the mentally impaired are taught what to expect when encountering such a client and how to deal with common problems.

1 2 3

ADMISSION

___ ___ ___ 6) A direct line representative of those staff who will be performing the care attend a pre-admission meeting to meet and assess the potential client.

___ ___ ___ 7) If an admission candidate is in hospital, a staff member visits or is in direct contact with the hospital to gain as much information as possible regarding the care process and routines already established.

___ ___ ___ 8) Where possible, the new admission and his/her family are gradually introduced to the unit prior to admission by establishing daily visits where meals and programs can be observed or participated in.

___ ___ ___ 9) Families are given an admission package outlining the specific needs of the mentally impaired, their role, philosophy of care for the mentally impaired client, programs involved, rights, etc.

____ 10) Families receive a questionnaire on admission asking them the client's preferences and care issues such as likes, dislikes, routines, abilities, how behavioral problems have been dealt with to this point, etc.

____ 11) The same staff are assigned to a new admission for the first three days to conduct the necessary assessment and develop the initial care plan.

____ 12) Only basic care is performed during the first few days of admission - bath, detailed assessment, activity involvement, etc. are withheld until the client gains familiarity with the unit and staff.

____ 13) During the first few days of admission, staff continually assess and respond to the client's need to be away from other clients and the routine of the unit.

____ 14) A meeting is held with family shortly after admission to adjust the care process.

____ 15) Potentially high risk clients are only admitted from hospital when a trial period can be negotiated with the referring agency guaranteeing the individual will be returned if he/she cannot be cared for safely within the facility.

1 2 3   **ENVIRONMENT**

____ 16) Environmental cueing (such as color coding and locator signs) are in place and each client is assessed to determine their ability to use each cue.

__ __ __ __ 17) Anchoring, the use of personal objects as locator cues (i.e. personal bedspread on their bed, specific decor on their door, etc.) is assessed and employed to assist the client to identify specific areas on the unit.

__ __ __ __ 18) The environment looks "normal", assisting the client to function by hooking "old memory" - dining room looks like a dining room, lounge like a living room, etc.

__ __ __ __ 19) There are areas available that allow the mentally impaired and cognitively well clients to be separate.

__ __ __ __ 20) There is a specific and clearly defined wandering path available to the mentally impaired clients.

__ __ __ __ 21) Exit doors accessible to the wanderer are secured with a locking system to allow the wanderer free and safe interior wandering.

__ __ __ __ 22) There is a secured courtyard that allows free access to the outside by all clients during appropriate weather conditions.

__ __ __ __ 23) Things familiar to the client's past are accessible in his/her room with the intention to "hook" old memories.

__ __ __ __ 24) All bedrooms housing the mentally impaired are private occupancy only.

__ __ __ __ 25) Multiple small sitting areas that are free from noise, stress and distraction are available (i.e. apart from the client's room).

_ _ _   26) Reality reinforcement supports are employed, where multiple cueing techniques (such as clocks, calendars, staff name tags, etc.) are assessed and appropriately located within the environment to help clients identify needed information.

1 2 3   **PROGRAMS**

_ _ _   27) Activity programs available to the mentally impaired are very distinct from programs available to other clients.

_ _ _   28) The recreation department maintains a list of mentally impaired clients and the programs each is involved in. All clients are regularly assessed regardless of their functioning ability, client participation rates and levels of participation are regularly monitored, evaluated and considered relative to program planning.

_ _ _   29) Sensory stimulation is employed by nursing, recreation and dietary department as an ongoing program.

_ _ _   30) There are well supervised and monitored large group activities for all mentally impaired clients encompassing all functioning stages of the disease process. The appropriateness of an individual participation in such activities is continually assessed.

_ _ _   31) There are a variety of small group activities geared to all functioning levels of client with mental impairment. One-to-one activities are scheduled, particularly for clients who cannot function well in a group setting

———— 32) There are regular outings specifically for all mentally impaired clients.

———— 33) Clients are continually assessed to determine what familiar and comforting therapeutic chores can be made available. These chores are geared to the individual's functioning level and can include cleaning glasses, setting tables, folding linen, etc.

———— 34) Activity equipment is available on the unit for any staff, volunteer or family to use at any time beyond the scheduled activity program. Guidelines are provided on how each activity is used for specific clients.

———— 35) Clients are actively involved and are given responsibility in the purchasing and daily care of plants in the facility.

———— 36) Pets are available to the mentally impaired. Clients are assessed to determine their role in providing pet care as a regular part of life and daily routines in the facility.

———— 37) Programming and events involving both clients and children are a normal routine in the daily lives of clients. Both clients and children engage in meaningful activities.

———— 38) Activity centers are available throughout the unit and visible to the wandering client (such as a rummaging room, writing desk, sewing and craft center, etc.). These centers are safe and designed to encourage the client to manipulate the available objects.

_ _ _ 39) Each department is responsible to monitor and develop programming for the mentally impaired clients in the building - nursing, recreation, housekeeping, restorative care, social services (where applicable), etc. All clients receive some form of regular programming regardless of the individual's functioning ability.

1 2 3   **CARE**

_ _ _ 40) Care giving and routines is flexible, and staff adjust their care in consideration of the circumstances and behavior encountered with a client at the time. Changes in routine are documented for possible integration into the client's care plan.

_ _ _ 41) Specific staff are responsible for a specific number of clients over a period of time, even though physical care on the unit may be completed as a team function. Assigned staff assume an advocate role, being actively involved in any care decisions for their assigned clients.

_ _ _ 42) All members of the care team (i.e. nursing, housekeeping, dietary and support staff, etc.) are actively involved in the care process and have input into the care practices of individual clients and the unit in general.

_ _ _ 43) Staff are involved in a process of care analysis (a formal mechanism to determine the causative factors behind any behavioral response) where everyone on the unit discusses the needs of each client and the best direction for care.

——— 44) Where possible, each full time staff has the same part time staff replacing him/her on the master schedule to provide consistent care giving.

——— 45) There is an up-to-date, accurate and effective care plan in place providing staff with the specifics of a client's routine, and guidelines on specific care practices for each client. The care plan is an integral part of care and is regularly adapted in response to the changing needs of the client.

——— 46) A detailed outline of the care plan accompanies any mentally impaired client transferred to hospital, along with the name of a facility contact person that hospital staff can call should problems in care occur.

——— 47) Family are considered an integral part of the care process, being informed of any changes in condition or care, and regularly empowered to augment the care provided.

——— 48) The care plan for the mentally impaired client is individualized and distinct from those involving the cognitively well clients, emphasizing psychological and behavioral issues as well as physical.

1 2 3   **ASSESSMENT**

——— 49) Assessments are conducted on admission, or when any noted change in a client's behavior or functioning ability occurs.

——— 50) All staff (RN, RNA, aides, recreation staff, housekeeping, dietary, etc.) are involved in the assessment process of any client and the collective sharing of results.

___ ___ ___   51) Staff understand the relationship between past history and present behavior. The assessment process requires staff to actively solicit and record information on the client's history, regardless of how long the person has lived in the facility.

___ ___ ___   52) A variety of functional assessment are completed on all clients at regular intervals. The value of the results are understood by direct staff and become an integral part of care and are included in the care plan.

___ ___ ___   53) The assessment process includes: functional assessment, mental status, medical, medication review, behavior and medication mapping, detailed history, environmental assessment and psychological profile.

___ ___ ___   54) Each client is assessed and reassessed as needed to determine the appropriateness of environmental cues used in the facility - name bars, color coding, shadow box, pictures, etc.

___ ___ ___   55) The process of ongoing informal assessment (observing subtle cues from a specific client in order to adjust care) is taught to all staff. Information uncovered is documented, integrated into the care plan and known by all staff in contact with the client, regardless of the department in which they work.

___ ___ ___   56) Clients who are chronically physically violent (beyond that which the facility is skilled to serve) - a threat to the safety of other clients and staff, despite intense efforts at assessment and behavior management - are transferred to a hospital or other specialized center for proper assessment or placement.

___ ___ ___   57) A procedure exists outlining the steps that must be taken to conduct a search when a client wanders from the building.

1 2 3   ## DRUGS & RESTRAINTS

___ ___ ___   58) Drugs are administered for client behavior only after other means are exhausted. When used, medications are viewed as an interim measure until alternative supportive measures can found.

___ ___ ___   59) A Three Month Drug Review is practiced requiring an automatic stop order on all drugs every three months, where each drug recorded is treated as a new order and the rationale for that drug written on the Doctor's Progress Notes.

___ ___ ___   60) Non-life maintenance drugs (sedations, sleeping pills, etc.) are subject to a trial period of decreased dosage or non-use when the initiating behavior is no longer obvious. It is the responsibility of all staff to monitor and communicate the results during the trial period.

___ ___ ___   61) All devices restricting the mobility of a client are considered   restraints (physical and chemical). A restraint policy exists requiring the team (including the physician) to decide whether any restraint is to be used on a specific client, and outlines precautions to be taken during the time the restraint is applied to the client. All clients (based on comprehension) and families are informed about the policy.

1 2 3   **STAFF**

___ ___ ___   62) All staff have been polled to identify those who do not wish to work with mentally impaired clients. These staff are not assigned to that level of care if at all possible.

___ ___ ___   63) Full and part time staff are consistently assigned to the same unit for a specific period of time, keeping to a minimum the number of different staff in contact with an individual client in any seven day period.

___ ___ ___   64) Staff in contact with the mentally impaired have been effectively trained to understand the diseases causing mental impairment, possible behaviors that may be encountered and the appropriate supportive measures and care strategies to be undertaken.

___ ___ ___   65) Staff responsible for the care of the mentally impaired clients have direct input into decision making regarding care, the environment in which the clients live and the programs affecting care.

___ ___ ___   66) There is a designated person or committee within the facility that has the responsibility to regularly monitor, evaluate and make recommendations on care practices for mentally impaired clients.

___ ___ ___   67) A staff member who has difficulty performing care with a specific client is not assigned that client. Training and support is provided to that staff member where appropriate. Instances where the client is a problem to a number of staff, or one staff member has problems with a number of clients, are dealt with individually.

— — —   68) A distinct support system exists for those staff working with the mentally impaired where time, break periods and routines can be adjusted in response to the events experienced on a specific day.

1 2 3   **FAMILY**

— — —   69) Family and significant others are considered part of the care process and are given the needed direction for their involvement in the care and activities of the client.

— — —   70) The facility has a family support group, allowing families the opportunity to meet with other families of mentally impaired clients, to learn about the disease process, programming options, the family's role and also provide family the chance to share with each other their feelings and experiences.

— — —   71) All family members of dementia clients (whether they are regular visitors or not) are referred to the local Alzheimer's Society for assistance and provided a list of available resource texts.

— — —   72) Families are notified in advance (through direct phone call, letter or a family bulletin board located in the facility) of any activities or outings scheduled for the mentally impaired clients, and families are encouraged to participate.

— — —   73) Families are provided the name of a contact person at a local social services agency to assist in dealing with the emotional issues that may arise through the course of the disease of their loved one.

_ _ _   74) The expertise of those families who have cared for a mentally impaired family member is recognized, and these families are encouraged to volunteer their services to assist in programs available in the building.

1 2 3   **VOLUNTEERS**

_ _ _   75) All volunteers are prepared for the possible behaviors they may encounter from the mentally impaired and the best approaches to be taken.

_ _ _   76) All available volunteers are polled to identify those who would like to work with the mentally impaired directly and in what capacity.

_ _ _   77) Volunteers who are asked to work with the mentally impaired receive ongoing training and follow-up to understand client behaviors and the most appropriate approaches to be taken.

_ _ _   78) All volunteers involved with the mentally impaired are "buddied" with the staff member who best knows the client in order to assist with any problems encountered.

1 2 3   **RESOURCES**

_ _ _   79) The care team has regular contacts with outside agencies and professionals for consultation when dealing with psychiatric and behavioral problems.

_ _ _   80) All members of the care team are encouraged to maintain their expertise by participating in training opportunities outside of the facility.

— — —

81) Staff development entails visits to other facilities involved in caring for the mentally impaired, to share and learn new skills and approaches.

— — —

82) The facility has a mandate and a means for the care team to share their accomplishments and expertise by submitting material to association publications or appropriate journals.

1 2 3

AUXILIARY PROGRAMS

— — —

83) A specialized Day Program is available within the facility for the mentally impaired living in the community, or if such a service exists outside the facility it is acknowledged and promoted.

— — —

84) A Respite or Vacation Care program for the mentally impaired living with family in the community is available within the facility and well promoted.

— — —

85) The facility is utilized as a resource center for family caring for mentally impaired individuals living in the community, encouraging them to call to gain information and assistance.

— — —

86) The facility has offered itself as a base for the local Alzheimer's Society or as a location to hold periodic meetings.

We are defining a specialty that is as challenging as any in the health care field. All of the practices and concepts presented are worthwhile and practical mechanisms for effectively caring for the mentally impaired clients with challenging behaviors. Your task is to decide which of these care components work well in your facility and which require implementation.

This is a developing industry and one that continues to evolve. The "magic" possessed by some individuals or some facilities in their success in caring for the mentally impaired is based totally on the energies they have invested to ensure such interventions are adapted to their environment and their resources.

Chapter Seventeen

Epilogue

Some ask, "How do you know that the world of the mentally impaired is as you described?" I don't! The challenge in this text has been to take a world of chaos and place it into logical terms. There is no way to be accurate in what is described. All that we can do is attempt to understand that person's world in whatever way possible. The closer we can come to the experience, the more effective our care will be.

This is not an exact science. Nothing we do in the health care field can be measured and dissected to clearly paint the whole picture of what each individual experiences when in such a crisis. Ours is a profession that is based on professional hunches. An attempt to pin down some direction. If it were easy there would be no challenge.

We have only begun to understand the mentally impaired. Their world is still a mystery, but the key to unlock that mystery is in view. The fear is that before we find a cure for Alzheimer's disease, we will find a way to slow it down rather than stop it. That may be a blessing to those mentally impaired who are in level one, still able to function, losing only minimal cognitive functioning. Those in level two, in conflict with reality, living in two worlds at the same time, dependent on others; and level three, those totally out of contact with reality and who can respond only to custodial care may not be so fortunate. The ability to medically slow the disease will raise some serious moral and ethical questions - do we take measures to have a person live twenty years with the disease by the treatment devised, or do we let the disease run its course, where the person will live only eleven years? There will be no easy answer, but a dilemma we will certainly face.

We will see further specialization in our field - becoming the "experts" in caring for the mentally impaired elderly. Either we prepare for our role now in a conscious effort to develop our resources and staff for this clientele, or we prepare for it when we are struck full force with the need.

There are some exciting things happening and some very skilled and creative individuals making them occur. No matter what you do, you are probably breaking new ground. No matter what you do, you are a pioneer in determining the best direction to care for the mentally impaired.

There will be struggles and battles that must be won to tap further resources. There will be a need to change many philosophies on the approach to be taken with this clientele. Ardently, you can be the main force in that change. I hope that this book has provided you with some guidance and direction in your quest to develop the best quality of life for this very special population. Beyond the specific suggestions, I have attempted to challenge you to be creative, to take chances in seeking new avenues towards better care. Go ahead. Accept the challenge - your initiative is needed and will make a difference.

Dance with grace and enjoyment! Your partner relies on you to stay in step.

Addendum

The following documents are contained within the addendum.

- Care Plan Summary
- Behavioral Incident Assessment
- Family Admission Questionnaire
- 24 Hour Profile

Care Plan Summary

Resident: _____   **Room Number:** _____

Base Line Data: Identify specific care requirements in each of these areas; expand on any pertinent data or specific approaches in the *Need to Know* section.

Toileting	_____	Bathing	_____
Dressing	_____	Teeth/Dentures	_____
Transfer	_____	Glasses	_____
Mobility	_____	Other	_____
Mealtime	_____	Other	_____

Stressor Profile: Identify triggers to be avoided for this resident i.e. noise, other residents, etc.

Daily Log: Identify exact times for daily routines/schedules i.e. waking time, care tasks, sits, wanders, activities, naps, bedtime, etc.

Time	Routine	Time	Routine

Need to Know: Identify important care issues and approaches for this resident (be specific and detailed) *Include:* What to talk about or do to distract. What not to talk about or do that will distress. How to approach. What to expect from this resident. Cues that indicate the resident is distressed or warning signs of impeding challenging behaviors. *(Use back of page if needed)*

_____

_____

_____

Behavioral Incident Assessment (Acute, LTC, Community, Family)

Date: _____

Time Behavior Witnessed: _____

Client's Name: _____

Behavior Observed: _____

Completed By: _____

Caregiver(s) Witnessing _____
    the Episode:

Complete the following assessment on the most recent incident.

- Describe in detail the actions of the client during the incident in question (what the client did or said).

- Did the client direct the behavior towards anyone or anything specifically: Yes No

    If Yes, identify the person(s) or thing(s)?

- Identify what was going on around or to the person at that time.

- Who was in contact with or around the client when the behavior occurred?

- Where was the client and what was the client doing prior to the incident?

- How long did the behavioral response last?

- What was the client like after the incident in question?

- What did the client do after the incident in question and where did the client go?

- Identify anything different about the environment, the individual's routine, medication used, etc. at the time or on the day of the incident.

- Identify how the situation could have been handled differently.

Family Admission Assessment

Family are to complete this form on admission to the best of their ability and then have it reviewed by staff to add any further details.

Meals: Likes and dislikes? What will your relative eat if they refuse everything else? What will your relative never eat? When is your relatives main meal? What are normal meal times? How much does your relative eat at each meal? What problems have you had getting your relative to eat? Any special arrangements or utensils used during meal time? Does your relative snack during the day (if yes, what)?	
Dressing: What can your relative do for himself regarding dressing and undressing? What does your relative need help with?	

Do you have any problems dressing or undressing your relative (if yes, what and how do you deal with it)? Is there anything your relative enjoys wearing more than others?	
Toileting: How do you know when your relative has to go to the bathroom? Are they incontinent? - if so, are they cooperative when you change them? Is there a pattern, special times or manner that helps you deal with toileting? Are there any medication or foods taken to assist with your relatives bowels?	
Bathing: Does your relative normally have a bath or shower? What time of day? Any problems in bathing? Special precautions or arrangements? Would you be willing to be present during your relatives first bath or two after admission?	

Problems combing and washing hair? Problems with mouth care? Does your relative brush their own teeth or do you do it for them?	
Ambulation: Does your relative wander? - if yes, when and how long? Is there a time of the day when you need to have your relative sit so they do not become over tired? What type of shoes does your relative wear? Does your relative use any walking aids - cane, railing, walker, etc.?	
Activities: What activities have you found your relative enjoys now? What activities did your relative do in the past that they no longer do? How long can your relative participate at an activity? What is the best time for your relative to do activities? Do you take them on outings? - if yes, where, when and how long?	

What do you talk about? Does your relative watch TV or listen to music? - if yes, what type? How often do you plan to visit? Who plans to visit? Are you willing to assist with activities or outings? - if yes, which day and time is most convenient?	
Sleeping: What time do they go to bed? Is your relative up during the night (how often)? Does your relative sleep during the day (when & how long)? Anything special about your relatives bed or room (personal quilt, number of pillows, light on, etc.)? When your relative wakes at night, how is their mental state? **Normal Day:** Describe a normal day for your relative. When are their "bad times"? How do you deal with those times?	

When would we know that your relative is getting anxious or agitated? Do you have any problems getting your relative to take their medication? Any special preparations for taking medications? What things does your relative find comforting? Is there a time of day that seems worse? How does your relative relate to new people?	
Understanding Your Relative: Describe your relative to me twenty years ago. How has your relative dealt with stress all of their life? What event(s) stand out in your relatives life?	

The 24 Hour Profile Questionnaire

This is a solutions oriented assessment. DO NOT expand on the care issues (problems or concerns) encountered. Provide only successful strategies employed or information known. The goal of this information is to:

1) Identify changes in functioning noticed between shifts (days, afternoons and nights).
2) Identify the client's strengths and limitations.
3) Identify successful techniques or approaches employed by certain staff in each area.

Step 1

This questionnaire is to be initiated by a staff member who best knows the client to be assessed. That staff member is required to complete the Supportive Data section for the shift that she has most contact with this client (day, evening or night shift). Be as specific as possible, recording any supportive data you believe appropriate to describe this individual's functioning in each area. In the space under Supportive Data include the following:

- pattern of behavior (time of day, equipment to be set in a specific manner, specific items used, etc.).
- when have you seen changes (will or will not function)?
- what do you say or do to assist the person to function?
- how can you tell if the individual is being pressured and it is best not to attempt the task at this time?

Step 2

The completed form is then reviewed by each shift (day, evening and night), adding to the information provided.

Step 3

Once completed, a list of care issues is extracted, and the guidelines outlined in the Supportive Data section providing the basis for the care plan.

24 Hour Profile

Resident Being Assessed

_____

Initial Assessment Completed By

_____

Date Of Initial Assess. _____

Date Reviewed _____

By Day Shift _____

Evening Shift _____

Night Shift _____

Supportive Data

ACTIVITIES OF DAILY LIVING	Yes	No	Day Shift	Evening/Night Shift
1. MEALTIME				
- needs assistance (explain)	( )	( )		
- easily distracted (how is this dealt with?)	( )	( )		
- can only handle few items at a time (which & in what order?)	( )	( )		
- any special arrangement or items?	( )	( )		
2. HYGIENE				
a) Bathing				
- co-operative in tub (if no, explain)	( )	( )		
- needs assistance (explain)	( )	( )		
- any special arrangements or items?	( )	( )		
b) Teeth/Hair				
- needs assistance (explain)	( )	( )		
- requires articles to be handed to him/her	( )	( )		
- cooperative during procedure (if no, explain)	( )	( )		
- any special arrangements or items?	( )	( )		
c) Dressing				
- requires assistance dressing or undressing (explain)	( )	( )		
- requires articles displayed	( )	( )		

	Yes	No	Supportive Data Day Shift	Evening/Night Shift
- requires articles to be handed to him/her	( )	( )		
- problems with specific articles of clothing	( )	( )		
- can pick own clothing from closet	( )	( )		
- any special arrangements or items?	( )	( )		

d) Toileting
- specific times (which?) ( ) ( )
- needs to be checked (when?) ( ) ( )
- how does he/she
    communicate the need to
    go to the washroom? (tell
    you or by what actions?) ( ) ( )
- any special arrangements or
    items? ( ) ( )

3. AMBULATION
- gait unsteady (describe) ( ) ( )
- needs to be checked, will
    exhaust self (what time of
    day and what is done if
    unsteady?) ( ) ( )
- wanders (identify time and
    specific area) ( ) ( )
- how do you deal with the
    wandering? ( ) ( )

4. COMPREHENSION
- understands instructions (if
    no, explain) ( ) ( )
- responds to his/her name
    (first, last or nickname?) ( ) ( )
- can identify staff or family
    members (who and how
    often?) ( ) ( )
-can identify all objects (if no,
    what and when?) ( ) ( )

	Yes	No	Supportive Data	
			Day Shift	Evening/Night Shift
-find way around unit - room, washroom, dining room, lounge, etc.	( )	( )		
-what must you do to help this person understand what you are saying or what you want done ?	( )	( )		

5. BEHAVIOR
In each area where (yes) is checked describe what the resident does and how you deal with it

	Yes	No		
-restless	( )	( )		
-repetitive behavior	( )	( )		
-destructive	( )	( )		
-disturbing behavior (to who?)	( )	( )		
-hoarding (what, from where?)	( )	( )		
-verbally/physically threatening others	( )	( )		

6. SOCIAL SKILLS

	Yes	No		
-can relate to others (will talk to who, when and about what?)	( )	( )		
-will help others (who and when?)	( )	( )		
-relates well to new people (if no, explain what happens)	( )	( )		
-participates in group activities (what and when?)	( )	( )		

	Yes No	<u>Day Shift</u>	<u>Evening/Night Shift</u>

7. ACTIVITIES

- will perform specific chores on the unit (what and when?) ( ) ( )

-be involved in specific games, hobbies (what, when and for how long?) ( ) ( )

- will read or look through books/magazines ( ) ( )

- enjoys music, TV (what and when?) ( ) ( )

Index